The Athletic Musician

A Guide to Playing without Pain

Barbara Paull

Christine Harrison

The Scarecrow Press, Inc.
Lanham, Md., & London
1997

SCARECROW PRESS, INC.

Published in the United States of America
by Scarecrow Press, Inc.
A wholly owned subsidiary of
The Rowman & Littlefield Publishing Group, Inc.
4501 Forbes Boulevard, Suite 200, Lanham, Maryland 20706
www.scarecrowpress.com

British Library Cataloguing in Publication Information Available

Library of Congress Cataloging-in-Publication Data

Paull, Barbara, 1936–
    The athletic musician : a guide to playing without pain / Barbara Paull,
Christine Harrison.
        p.   cm.
    Includes bibliographical references and index.
    ISBN 0-8108-3356-5 (pbk. : alk. paper)
    1. Musicians—Wounds and injuries.   I. Harrison, Christine, 1956– .
    RC965.P46P38   1997
    617.1'0088'78—dc21   97-20326

ISBN 0-8108-3356-5

Manufactured in the United States of America.

Contents

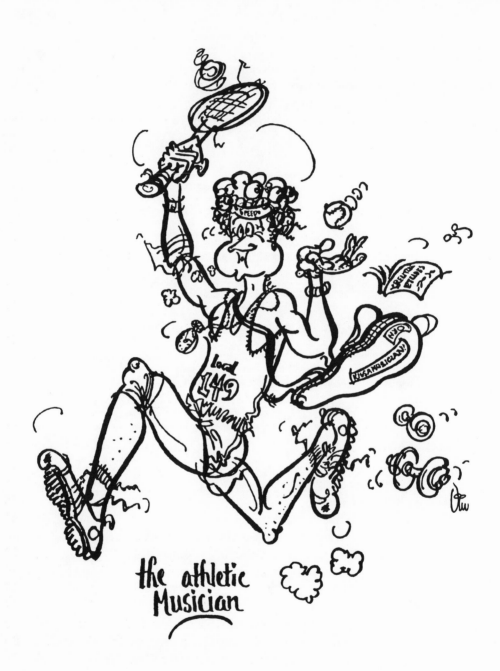

the athletic
Musician

Illustrations

Photographs, by Brian Harrison and Michael Paull

Foreword

Musicians are athletes capable of amazing feats of stamina and control, the likes of which would be the envy of professional sports men and women. They, like their instruments, have to be finely tuned. A less-than-optimal muscle balance or maintaining a posture for hours on end for which the body was not designed can wreak havoc.

This book is like a maintenance manual for an incredibly complex and sophisticated machine, the human body, showing how to keep it running smoothly and how to correct it when it is not. Although not a musician, apart from singing in the bath, I have some personal experience of the thinking behind the book.

For years I had pain in my shoulder when playing tennis. I tried various remedies, to no avail. I was fortunate enough to have my shoulder assessed by Barbara Paull. She demonstrated that I had about as much strength in my infraspinatus as a piece of stewed rhubarb. She suggested that I work on that. I did, and the muscle balance was restored. I have had no problems since.

The application of the principles so lucidly expressed in this book will undoubtedly save thousands upon thousands of hours of dysfunction and pain in musicians.

Michael A. Barnett, M.B., B.S., F.R.C.S.(Eng), F.R.C.S.(Can)
Orthopedic Surgeon
Poole, Dorset, England

Preface

The sports coach today is expected to have a reasonable knowledge about the workings of the athlete and how to assist this performer to achieve the highest output.

During the past few years it has been expected that coaches acquire qualifications which provide greater insight for developing the athlete's performance and safeguarding the athlete's welfare. Even without appropriate knowledge, the coach may have easy access to advisors who provide expertise about such important aspects as exercise prescription, strength and skill development, efficiency of movement and the prevention and management of injury. Psychologists are now regularly employed to provide that extra winning edge while sociologists and physiologists may be consulted to help with the identification of young potential talent. It would appear that the sports world has a distinct edge when compared to other spheres of life where the human body is subjected to continual physical stress. Furthermore, one sees sports medicine clinics in many localities, and medical doctors and physiotherapists are linked professionally with successful elite athletes. We are now beginning to see the need for musicians to be assisted in a similar fashion, but for an orchestra or musical ensemble to have an entourage of medical and movement specialists would be perceived as somewhat strange. A concert pianist or violinist with a personal physiotherapist in tow would seem logical, but would still be regarded as unusual.

Sport has enjoyed the added distinction of having its activities positively linked with health, and sporting teams have surrounded themselves with appropriate body experts. People in the performing arts, however, do not have that link.

Despite the perceived advantages that sports groups appear to enjoy, because the product (that is, winning) is often seen as more important than the process of playing, athletes may still be disadvantaged by being expected to perform despite injury, fatigue or illness. In these situations, the supposedly knowledgeable teacher may conveniently ignore obvious signs of athlete pain because the attraction of a winner is culturally more acceptable than a loser. Musicians may similarly be distracted by overt competition and there is still the implied requirement for an ensemble or individual to perform despite physical discomfort. It is hoped that appropriate physiotherapy support can become a normal part of orchestras, dance troupes and other performing arts groups. This book ably explains this need by strongly urging the key decision makers to look upon their performers also as athletes, and not merely as technicians who focus solely on fine motor skills, dexterity and musicianship. Health care expertise has an important contribution to make for performance areas beyond the playing field to concert platforms and theatrical stages.

Michael J. Reynolds, Ph.D.
Lecturer
School of Human Movement & Sports Sciences
University of Ballarat
Ballarat, Victoria, Australia

Acknowledgments

There are a great many people we would like to thank for their help in making this book possible.

Our thanks to three wonderful artists: Sara Beeton, medical illustrator (and violin maker), for her innovative anatomical drawings; Craig Sinclair, for the cover design, his diagrams and non-sexist exercise sketches; and Viiu Varik, an "athletic bass-playing musician" for inspiring our title with her portrayal of "The Athletic Musician."

Our thanks to Ashvin Karia of Photoland, Newmarket, for generously allowing us to take over his studio and equipment, and to Brenda Gottlieb, Piano Tuner and Technician, for her inside scoop on pianos.

Thanks to Gretchen Anner, who immediately incorporated our teaching into hers and provided a press photograph to prove it.

A number of willing victims posed for photographs, often having to pose in poor playing postures they wouldn't be caught dead in! Thanks to Hans Fischer, Robert Carlton, Lorraine Rousseau, Lutia Lausane, Anita Stern, Gary Macey, Suzanne Jung, Viiu Varik, Jonathan Paull, Susan Paull, Catherine Paull, Andrea Harrison, Daniel Harrison, and Brian Chatterton.

Special thanks to our long-suffering husbands, Michael Paull and Brian Harrison. Michael tolerated two computer illiterates and managed to put the book down on paper in spite of us. Brian and Michael both took photographs, generally did whatever needed doing, and are tied in first place for the "Helpful Husband" award.

PART 1

The Problem

Introduction

Listening to a symphony orchestra or watching a soloist perform, the uninitiated listener is aware only of the music that issues forth so effortlessly. The performers, of course, know that music-making doesn't just happen and that thousands of hours of practicing have gone into their "effortless" performance before they even get on the stage. But until they push themselves to the point of pain or loss of function, the musicians themselves often remain ignorant of the demands that playing makes upon their bodies.

Overuse injuries, which comprise the majority of musicians' injuries, are not a new phenomenon.[1] But until very recently we heard only of those isolated cases of high-profile performers who had to abandon their careers because of injury. In fact, musicians' injuries are a widespread, almost universal problem, affecting players of all levels in every instrument group.

Statistics on the prevalence of musicians' injuries vary widely, ranging from high to very high. Fishbein and Middlestadt's survey[2] of 2,212 ICSOM (International Conference of Symphony and Opera Musicians) members concludes that "76 percent of musicians performing . . . reported at least one medical problem that was severe in terms of its effect on performance." Even when one takes into consideration that these "medical problems" were not limited to musculoskeletal injuries, the following statistics from that survey are alarming, to say the least.

The conclusion to data listed in table I.1 is stated as "The findings clearly show a very high prevalence of medical problems in this population. Fully 76% of musicians performing with the 48 ICSOM orchestras reported at least one medical problem that was severe in terms of its effect on performance. . . . The neck and back were the most frequently mentioned locations for musculoskeletal problems. . . . Given the proportions of professional musicians reporting medical problems severe enough to affect performance, there can be little doubt that music medicine is a field that deserves serious attention from health professionals."

Injury problems appear across every section of the orchestra, with string players leading the way in the ICSOM survey (above) with 82 percent reporting

Table I.1. Some Highlights from the 1987 Survey of ICSOM Musicians

Problem	Location	Percent Mentioning as	
		Problem	Severe Problem
Finger	Right	9	5
Finger	Left	16	9
Hand	Right	9	5
Hand	Left	14	10
Wrist	Right	10	5
Wrist	Left	9	5
Forearm	Right	7	4
Forearm	Left	8	5
Elbow	Right	10	6
Elbow	Left	8	4
Shoulder	Right	**20**	**13**
Shoulder	Left	**20**	**11**
Neck	Right	**21**	**13**
Neck	Left	**22**	**12**
Upper Back	Right	16	9
Upper Back	Left	16	8
Middle Back	Right	11	5
Middle Back	Left	11	5
Lower Back	Right	**22**	**13**
Lower Back	Left	**22**	**11**

Reprinted with permission of Hanley and Belfus Inc.

at least one medical problem and 76 percent indicating at least one severe medical problem. In another 1986 survey of 250 professional musicians,[3] 57 percent reported musculoskeletal performance-related disorders, with 34 percent of performance-impaired musicians showing lost income as a result of these problems. No specific statistics are available on the incidence of injury among pianists and guitarists (neither of which are found in large numbers in orchestras!) but our own experience at the Stouffville Musicians' Clinic and the number of these injured musicians we speak to at our "Playing without Pain" workshops tell us that they are far from exempt from injury problems. Problems are not limited to adult professionals. In one survey, amateur musicians reported a 72 percent incidence of overuse injuries.[4] There are few statistics available on elementary school-aged children (again, we can report them as regular visitors to our clinic), but figures at the university level vary from 10-20 percent in one study of students in Australian music schools[5] to 87 percent of students at an American university reporting some degree of performance pain.[6] The data we can't collect is perhaps the most upsetting. We don't know how many young people have had to give up their dreams of a career in music because of injury problems, or how many professional players have had to drop out in mid-career.

Sound like a desperate, hopeless situation? We hope we can prove to you that it doesn't have to be that way. Musicians' injuries should not be ranked with other horrible, incurable diseases and conditions. The scientific knowledge to successfully prevent and treat the vast majority of playing injuries already exists.

Notes

1. Dr. B. Ramazzini in 1713 wrote that "No sort of exercise is so healthful or harmless that it does not cause serious disorders . . . when overdone."

2. Fishbein M, Middlestadt SE, Ottati V, et al.: Medical problems among ICSOM musicians: Overview of a national survey. *Med Probl Perform Art* 3:1-8, 1988.

3. Caldron PH, Calabrese LH, Clough JD, et al.: A survey of musculoskeletal problems encountered in high-level musicians. *Med Probl Perform Art* 1:136-39, 1986.

4. Newmark J, Lederman RJ: Practice doesn't necessarily make perfect: Incidence of overuse syndromes in amateur instrumentalists. *Med Probl Perform Art* 2:142-44, 1987.

5. Fry HJH: Prevalence of overuse (injury) in Australian music schools. *Br. J. Ind. Med.* 44:35-40, 1987.

6. Pratt RR, Jessop SG, Niemann BK: Performance-related disorders among music majors at Brigham Young University. *IJAM* 1(2):7-20, 1992.

Chapter 1

The Psychology of Musicians' Injuries

How did we get into this mess in the first place?

In the absence of research indicating that musicians are predisposed to masochism, we can say that most of us do not enjoy pain any more than the next fellow. Yet as a group we have come to accept pain and discomfort as an inevitable part of playing. It didn't take much to bring us around to this defeatist way of thinking, and every survey that brings new statistics to our attention reinforces our fatalistic attitude about our profession. Musicians are left wondering if we could get better insurance rates by switching to a safer occupation, like skydiving!

We know that a few of us manage to get through without any difficulties, but we don't understand why. Musicians are taught little, if anything, about anatomy and the principles of injury prevention. Because we have such limited understanding of how our bodies work when we play, every frightening statistic about the prevalence and severity of injuries feeds the myth of their inevitability. Our ignorance also means we are uneducated consumers and sitting ducks for any kind of inappropriate or dangerous treatment that comes along.

Complicating matters further is the fact that music-making is likely one of the last areas of endeavor where the "no pain no gain" myth still reigns. Perhaps some of us are aware that this has been scientifically proven to be false, but on an emotional level most of us still fall into the trap of believing that pain is a component of excellence. Well-intentioned but misguided teachers are often among the first influences in our acceptance of this myth, admonishing students not to use the "excuse" of pain to curtail their work, and teaching them that the "harder" they work and the more they exhaust themselves, the greater the progress. How many musicians feel that a good practice session is one that leaves you looking for a crowbar to pry your exhausted and stiffened body away from the instrument? Our mind -set of "success at any cost" feeds this myth, and results in many of us thinking that to be pain-free means we must sacrifice progress or quality in our music-making.

Medical professionals can unwittingly reinforce the musicians' belief that they must play in pain when they fail to provide a long-term solution to an injury problem and instead manage recurring symptoms with "Band-Aid" treatments. We get the same message when an extended "rest" is prescribed. This puts musicians in a "no win" situation. Both emotionally and financially, injured players probably can't stay away from their careers for months or years and if they continue to play they will continue to hurt or, worse yet, get to the point where they are unable to play at all. It's little wonder that so many players stay away from orthodox medicine altogether,[1] preferring to muddle through on their own, putting up with discomfort and pain, or seeking temporary relief from their symptoms through "alternatives" to medicine.

In the chapters to come, you'll read about my own struggle with an injury that nearly ended my career. Horror stories like mine abound, usually minus the happy ending. The common thread in all our experiences is not just what happens to us, but why and how it happens. Looking back, most of us will find that we ran into trouble because of:

    a. our ignorance of the demands playing makes on our body
    b. our acceptance of pain as a part of music-making
    c. our justifiable paranoia about our reputation and job security, which
        often prevents us from seeking help

And when we go for help we encounter a medical profession that seldom understands what's involved in being a musician, which often results in:

    d. ineffective, inappropriate, and sometimes dangerous treatment, and
    e. musicians who continue to play hurt

It is not surprising that so many musicians believe that the best they can expect is a life-long dependency on treatments which, while they never get to the root of the problem, keep their symptoms under control to a degree that they can at least continue to play and work, albeit with discomfort and/or pain.

So often the tragedy is not that successful treatment is unavailable or that injuries cannot be prevented, but that musicians have been convinced by their own experiences and those of others that nothing can be done for them. We hope that by reading this book you will learn about the underlying causes of musicians' injuries and scientifically sound principles of prevention and treatment. Armed with this knowledge, you'll begin to rethink what you do and how you do it and no longer settle for anything less than comfortable, pain-free playing.

Note
1. Only 21 percent of pain-affected music students surveyed at Brigham Young University sought help from a physician (Pratt RR, Jessop SG, Niemann BK: Performance-related disorders among music majors at Brigham Young University. *IJAM* 1(2):7-20, 1992).

Chapter 2

A Physiotherapist's Opinion

As a physiotherapist I find it incredibly sad that music, which uplifts and sustains the human spirit, can simultaneously cause pain and injury for musicians. After thirty years of practicing orthopedic physiotherapy, I am also firmly convinced that musicians' injuries are no different from those suffered by elite athletes and many dedicated workers. Their problems are best described as soft tissue injuries, meaning hurt muscles, tendons, ligaments, nerves and discs, none of which show on x-rays. They can cause sufficient pain and weakness or changes in normal sensation in the hands to make it impossible for a musician to play. Yet all of these soft tissues are designed to work hard and, like all joints in the body, deteriorate with immobility.

Both musicians and athletes place tremendous demands upon their bodies, practicing their skills for many hours and stressing themselves physically and psychologically in competition and in pursuit of excellence. Discounting athletes engaged in contact or high-risk sports, it seems fair to compare musicians with ball players, swimmers or track and field eventers. All are involved in hard, repetitive, physical work and are under constant pressure to perform well.

That is where the similarities stop. Competitive athletes are under the eagle eyes of athletic coaches whose job it is to ensure that athletes are generally fit and in good physical condition, as well as practicing their sports using protocols designed to protect them from physical harm. Sports psychologists are available to nurture their well-being and to teach them body-saving techniques such as mental practicing and visualization. Musicians, on the other hand, simply learn to play. Their teachers have little knowledge of the effects of repeated exercise or sustained postures upon the body, other than commonsense responses to their own injuries. In fact, some music teachers, frequently playing in pain themselves, may help perpetuate the myth that pain is a necessary part of becoming an accomplished musician.

Nothing could be further from the truth. Pain is the only way the body can tell you that it is being hurt or damaged and it is trying to get your attention so that you will do something about it. To accept or ignore pain, or to play through it, is inviting disaster.

Musicians need a whole new area of knowledge. First, they need to perceive themselves as musical athletes, then they need to know how to look after their bodies and avoid playing injuries. Last of all, musicians need to know simple, self-help techniques to combat the first sign of any familiar aches or pain at sites of common musicians' injuries—and where to go for help if these pains do not immediately respond to self-treatment.

Grading the Severity of Overuse Playing Injuries (OPI)

Using a scale similar to that used in the Clinic to grade worker's injuries, musicians' injuries can be graded thus:

Grade I	Pain occurs after playing, but the musician can still perform normally.
Grade II	Pain occurs during playing, but the musician's performance is not restricted.
Grade III	Pain occurs during playing and the musician has to alter the playing position or curtail performance.
Grade IV	Pain occurs as soon as the musician attempts to play and is too severe to continue.
Grade V	Pain is continuous, during all activities of daily living. Playing is out of the question.

Grade I injuries generally respond to education and ergonomic advice. Grades II through V usually need some physiotherapy treatment as well. The short-term goal is to give rapidly effective, localized treatment to the injury and the long-term goal is to prevent recurrence of that or any other injury by teaching the musical athletes all they need to know so they will not require further treatment.

No athlete, musical or otherwise, should have to depend upon frequent or repetitive treatments of any description. Our bodies are amazingly forgiving and have great recuperative powers. We heal, often despite ourselves. Torn muscles heal in about four weeks. Sprained ligaments heal in about six weeks. The majority of neck and back strains are better in six to eight weeks, as is acute tendonitis, unless all are continually being re-injured or irritated. Even if one breaks the biggest bone in one's body, the thigh bone, it is expected to heal in about twelve weeks. Injuries do not go on forever and acute soft tissue injuries should start to improve noticeably within one month, unless the tissue abuse continues.

In the following chapters we will present a case history of Christine Harrison's experience following a serious playing injury, typical for a professional violinist. We will then describe the reasons for this and other musicians' injuries, looking at simplified layman's anatomy and physiology to explain the sequence of events from a vague ache or tingle to severe pain or numb fingers.

Finally, we will present athletic protocols appropriate for musicians, addressing on- and offstage activities to keep you playing without pain. If you are already hurt, this book is in no way a replacement for the specific help and advice of your own orthopedic physiotherapist.

Chapter 3

The Musician's Tale

In the fall of 1983 I was starting my professional career, playing violin in an opera company orchestra. I was in my second season of professional freelancing in Toronto, a well-trained, relaxed player in the early stages of what promised to be a successful career as an orchestral musician. I had never had any injury problems and was totally unaware that being a musician could be dangerous to your health. But within a space of two months, everything changed. I found myself in constant pain and scarcely able to move my right arm. For the next four years I struggled unsuccessfully to return to playing, as my hopes and dreams of being a violinist crumbled with each passing year. But like any good fairy tale, there is a happy ending. I've been playing pain-free since 1987. So let me tell you about what went on between "once upon a time" and "happily ever after."

How It All Started (September 1983)

Playing second violin in a Wagner opera ranks at the top of the list of how to live dangerously as a violinist. There are few things in our career that are as grueling (Paganini caprices and off-beats for Strauss waltzes coming a close second and third!). Being the "new kid on the block" and a perfectionist at heart, I was putting in a few hours of practice every day on top of services two hours longer than I was used to, during the two-week run of the opera. I don't remember feeling any "pain" at the time – just fatigue and a nagging sense of being increasingly uncomfortable. But having relived the onset of my symptoms of injury ad nauseam, in retrospect I can pinpoint the warning signs that should have made the lights go on. Fatigue after hard work is normal. As musicians, we are performing an activity that is physically demanding and we can expect to be tired after working hard. But when you're feeling fatigued during the overture, you know you're in trouble. I found that it took an enormous effort to lift my right arm. Playing on the lower strings (with my arm in its most elevated position) was exhausting. While I wasn't aware of severe pain at this time, I did feel a little "grab" as I tried to raise my arm, and again as I tried to lower it. I

11

compensated subconsciously by tilting my violin more (a trick every violist knows). I raised my shoulder with every bow stroke and kept my right elbow as low as I could.

Injuring myself was amazingly easy, decidedly undramatic, and took absolutely no special effort on my part. All I had to do was what almost everyone of us has done at some point in their career. I worked a little harder than I was used to without understanding anything about my body's involvement in my playing. And of course, being a musician means putting up with discomfort and pain, so I ignored all my body's warning signals in the name of "dedication" to what I was doing. I kept on going until gradually every part of my body felt uncomfortable as I limped along, trying to compensate for what I thought was my sore arm.

Back in those days before people were talking about musicians' injuries, I had no idea you could hurt yourself "just" playing the violin. At that time my only acquaintance with the whole subject of injuries was a vague concept of "tendonitis." I assumed that I had a touch of tendonitis in my right arm and that it would settle on its own when the opera run finished and I took a break. Wrong!

I developed a career-threatening injury, not because I worked harder than the next person or because I enjoyed pain. Like the majority of musicians' injuries, mine was not the result of some trauma. (Despite what doctors tried to tell me, I have no recollection whatsoever of swinging from chandeliers, throwing my arm out of the socket pitching for the Blue Jays baseball team, or getting hit by a truck.) My injury happened because I worked hard at something I loved to do, because I was ignorant of what was going on with my body, and because I had the typical musicians' acceptance of the "no pain, no gain" myth. These are the factors that conspired to lead me down the road to injury. And what a long road it turned out to be! I had absolutely no idea that this little problem would in fact threaten my career, and that the closing night of the opera would mark the last time I'd play professionally for five years.

With the mistaken notion that I was doing the right thing, I took a complete break for two weeks when the opera ended, and then resumed playing. When my arm felt tired instantly despite my vacation, I put it down to a bit of stiffness because I hadn't played for a while. When it still felt tired and started to ache a few weeks down the road, I thought it was perfectly normal because I was practicing a lot. When it started to feel like I needed a winch to get my arm up to the lower strings, I suspected that maybe I did have just a touch of tendonitis. When the little "grabs" turned into serious pain, I told myself that when I had time perhaps I should do something about it. When I was sitting down and tried to reach something on the table in front of me and found that I couldn't lift my hand off my lap, I finally admitted that maybe I had a problem.

Looking for Help (November 1983 - February 1986)

My first step was a visit to my family doctor who took a very conservative line of treatment. He told me that my problem originated in the shoulder and suggested that I take a week off from playing. He recommended ice to reduce the inflammation and treated the pain with acupuncture. When a week had passed without much improvement, he prescribed an anti-inflammatory drug. Acupuncture treatments helped to relieve the pain. After two weeks I felt better and could move more and I carefully resumed playing. But within a few days of moderate playing, I found myself back at square one, with so much pain and so little movement that I couldn't play. Put repeat signs around this paragraph, mark it "vamp" and you've got the story of what the next four years of my life were like.

Each time I tried to play and found I couldn't, I would go to a highly qualified medical practitioner, including many physiotherapists, a massage therapist, neurologists and four orthopedic surgeons. They would take a history and conduct various tests to arrive at their diagnoses. These tests included x-raying my shoulder so many times that I thought it would glow in the dark, sending electrical currents down my arm to see if I was short-circuiting somewhere (EMG) and yanking my arm away from my body and measuring how far I jumped off the examining table.

Every medical professional I saw arrived at a conclusion. The difficulty lay in the fact that all the conclusions were different. Diagnoses given included tendonitis, bursitis, arthritis, a pinched nerve in my neck, a dislocating shoulder, possible thoracic outlet syndrome, adhesive capsulitis and a disinserted long head of the biceps. Ultimately, I was given medicine's standard answer to unsolved problems – I was crazy and had dreamed the whole thing up because I didn't really want to be a musician.

Treatments varied as much as the diagnoses, the only common factor being the recommendation to rest. I was told to abstain from playing for periods of time varying from my family doctor's sensible suggestion of a week, to an orthopedic surgeon's recommendation of six months. Meanwhile, I was given every anti-inflammatory medication on the market. After three years of popping pills that did nothing other than give me stomach problems, I decided that if I couldn't play I would at least like to be able to eat and refused further prescriptions. A bag of frozen vegetables made a cheap, effective anti-inflammatory and the only side-effect was a lasting aversion to peas!

Some treatments gave me temporary relief from pain, with acupuncture being the most effective. Two years of massage therapy also made me feel better for short periods of time, but didn't help resolve my problem. All that time and money spent on massage treatments wasn't wasted – my masseur developed great muscles and I learned how to give great back rubs.

My sensible family doctor suggested physiotherapy as the first line of defense when two weeks of treatment with him hadn't eliminated the problem. He had the right idea, but unfortunately the hospital had a six-month waiting list and the private physiotherapist I went to took a very passive approach to the problem and never figured out what had caused it in the first place. I spent a few months going for treatments which consisted of stretches, exercises, ultrasound, heat, ice, etc., all to no avail.

Three years down the road, I tried physiotherapy again, this time at the recommendation of an orthopedic surgeon. He felt that my difficulties stemmed from poor upper body development. After three years of not being able to use my right arm I had no muscle left, although I questioned how this could have been responsible for the onset of my injury as at that time I had been able to play for seven or eight hours a day. This second course of physiotherapy involved all the usual things, as well as extensive upper-bodybuilding. Three days a week, for two hours at a time, I worked out at a fitness center, under the supervision of a large group of "therapists." When I asked them why I could do 25-lb. biceps curls and couldn't raise my arm from my side without pain, they told me to keep working at it. After three months of bodybuilding I still couldn't play. By this point, I had dismissed physiotherapy as (a) time consuming, (b) ineffective and (c) costly. Apart from the actual treatment costs, there was the expense of replacing all my blouses I could no longer fit into.

Whenever I completed a course of therapy, the person directing my treatment would tell me that I "should" be able to play, but every time I started to play, I ended up in pain. Sometimes the pain would come back after only a few minutes of playing. Sometimes I could last for 30 minutes, but woke up the next day unable to move my upper arm. If I got to the third day and could still play, I thought I might be out of the woods. One time I made it all the way to four days, which made the crash even worse when it inevitably arrived.

Four years was a long time to spend going back to square one and I was getting desperate. Doctors couldn't give me any explanation for my condition, but told me that the only chance I had of resuming my career would be to bow with my left hand or take up the cello. Without a plausible explanation for my problem, I couldn't give up hope that someday I'd be able to play again. After a lot of careful thought, with advice from several medical professionals, I took what I believed to be the last option available to me. With the aim of having someone actually look into the shoulder joint and find out once and for all what was going on, I consented to an exploratory arthroscopic operation. Big mistake!

The Operation (February 1986)

Even though "desperate" certainly describes my frame of mind at the time, I did not consent to surgery without careful consideration. The problem lay in the fact that the advice I was given came from surgeons – and "to someone with a hammer, everything looks like a nail."

"Dr. X" who performed my surgery was very eminent in his field and had impeccable credentials. I had several consultations with him before going through with the operation. His theory was that I was suffering from a "baseball" shoulder, the result of strenuous overhand pitching. (I don't play baseball.) He wanted to put stainless steel pins in the shoulder joint to keep it from dislocating. When I asked him if that would enable me to return to playing the violin, he said that he thought it "should," giving me odds of 50-50. I wasn't entirely convinced that adding hardware to my shoulder was the answer, so we agreed that he would check things out first. He wanted to confirm his diagnoses by putting me under anesthetic and then seeing how easily he could make my shoulder pop in and out of the socket. He also wanted to look into the joint with an arthroscope to get a better idea of what was going on. He presented this surgery to me as a simple 20-minute operation that would leave me with no ill effects other than three minuscule scars on my shoulder and a few hours of discomfort. He described the surgery as "noninvasive," which should have been my cue to head for the nearest exit. I headed instead to the operating room, not looking forward to the surgery, but very anxious to discover what had happened to my shoulder and find out once and for all whether or not I'd ever play again. I signed a consent form for surgery on this understanding, having read it carefully and in fact crossing out the provision that an intern be allowed to operate, wanting only the prestigious Dr. X to perform the procedure.

My first clue that things had not gone according to plan came when I looked at the clock in the recovery room. The nurses confirmed that my 20-minute operation had actually lasted an hour longer than planned. Then Dr. X came to speak with me. My first question was, of course, "Will I be able to play?" When he answered "Play? Play what?" my heart sank and I knew I was in deep trouble. He proceeded to tell me that I wasn't going to be a candidate for the next bionic woman as my shoulder was not "frankly dislocating," but that the joint was in a terrible mess. While I was under anaesthetic and seeing as he was already in there with the arthroscope, he did me the favor of "cleaning up" the shoulder at the same time. It was quite a job, he said, as there were a lot of things that needed snipping, tidying up and rearranging. As a matter of fact, some of it was looking rather worn, so he removed it for me. I have a hand-written note from Dr. X to my family doctor, giving instructions on removal of the stitches, and explaining that he removed part of the labrum. My family doctor wasn't pleased that Dr. X had done me this favor while I was under anesthetic. A few weeks after the operation when he requested a complete copy of my file, he was told that it was "lost." I do have a copy of a letter from Dr. X to the referring orthopedic surgeon. This letter describes somebody's operation and treatment plan – not mine. There was no explanation given for the cause of the condition of the joint. There was no recommendation for further treatment other than a few Tylenol and the suggestion that I stop on the way home and pick up a coil chest-expander exerciser to start working with the next day.

The next day found me unable to open the box the exerciser came in and the Tylenol didn't touch the pain. Two weeks later I still hurt and I couldn't move my arm at all. I wasn't just back at square one — I wasn't even on the board any more.

The Beginning of the End (March 1986)

It was only out of desperation and at the insistence of my family doctor that I agreed to go to yet another physiotherapist, but I knew immediately that Barbara was different from the rest. She began by asking for a history, which I gave starting with the operation and working back through all the various things I had tried. Barbara was so upset at what she heard that before I could finish she put her hands up and said "Stop — I can't listen to any more." She started treatment for the postsurgical mess she found me in, explaining that before anything else could happen we had to restore full movement to the shoulder joint. Treatments were very painful, but I could see the progress I made with each visit. I was given various stretches and exercises to do at home and within a period of a few months I was able to move my arm normally again.

Unlike any other health care professional I had dealt with, Barbara's top priority was getting me back to playing, even though by this point I had almost given up hope. Barbara never told me that I "should" be able to play. Instead, she said, "Christine, you can start playing again." After I got off the floor, she explained to me that now that I had full motion and no pain, the only missing ingredient was strength. But the shoulder joint was still very "irritable" and conventional strengthening exercises made it flare up. Since I wanted to regain my strength so I could play the violin, she reasoned that I should use playing itself as my strengthening exercise. Barbara had already taught me that playing an instrument was an athletic activity, not just an artistic one, and concluded my treatment with some advice about how to "train." We discussed practice schedules and she advised me to start by timing my sessions and limiting them to five minutes a day. I "graduated" from physiotherapy and Barbara sent me on my way with her sincere wishes for my success, combined with the admonishment that I'd better take it easy and remember what she'd taught me because she never wanted me to darken the door of her clinic again. (Little did she know.)

I floated home on cloud nine, dusted off the violin case and then panicked. I had waited for this moment for so long, but once I was faced with the reality of picking up my violin again, I was scared to death. I was afraid that my body would let me down. I still didn't really understand what had caused the whole problem, so I thought there might be something inherently wrong with me that would make another injury inevitable. I was afraid to take the chance of having my hope destroyed again – I didn't think I could withstand another crash. Even without any injury recurrence, I knew that it would take a long time to regain my skills as a violinist and I was afraid that I wouldn't be able to do it.

If I'd looked at things logically, I probably would have shut the case and spent my energy trying to sue Dr. X. If I'd looked at things logically, I likely would never have chosen to be a violinist in the first place, so fear and logic took a back seat, hope and determination kicked in, and I played.

Getting Back in Shape (Summer 1986 - Summer 1987)

I was in a unique position at this time. My body felt as if I'd never played before, but mentally I had the ability of a professional violinist. I knew what I wanted to do and how to do it, but getting my body to cooperate was another story. Picking up the instrument in these circumstances gave me a new perspective on playing. Like any other well-taught player, I knew a lot about right and left hand positions, but now I realized how much the entire body was involved in playing. I discovered how merely holding the violin necessitates positions that are unnatural, but feel normal to us only because we've been in them for so long. I was also made acutely aware of which aspects of playing are strenuous and fatiguing. I knew no one else who had been in this unusual situation before, so I had to work things out for myself. Drawing on what Barbara had taught me, I had to rethink everything about playing and practicing from the viewpoint of an athlete, using past experience as a player, mixed with basic common sense about what would work for me.

Barbara need not have worried about my doing too much too soon. My first practice session after the operation lasted less than my prescribed five minutes – I could not hold my arm up for that long. For the first while it took me twice as long to warm up and stretch as it did to practice, but over the next year I gradually built up strength and endurance. At the beginning of my "recovery" year, it was difficult to believe that I would ever regain my skills as a violinist. As a well-known violinist once said, "If I miss one day of practicing, I can tell; if I miss two days, everyone can tell." After four years off, I think our dog could tell.

Despite the fact that I hadn't played for so long or consciously even thought about playing, I found that I had a much clearer picture of what I wanted to do. At some level of consciousness I must have been incubating ideas that were just waiting for a chance to come to fruition, and in many ways I believe that I ended up a better player because of what had happened to me. (This is not intended as a recommendation to hurt yourself ! There must be an easier way.)

One device that helped me during those early stages was setting goals, starting with my first goal of making it to the five-minute bell, to my final goal of playing the Bach "Chaconne" twice in a row (which I had never attempted while healthy). I was not interested in being able to play in a limited way. I wanted to be able to play better than I had before, without any limitations, or I wouldn't play at all. Because I had been disappointed so many times, I made a deal with myself that if I could pass the "Bach" test, then it would be safe to believe that I had fully recovered.

I reneged on the deal. Now I could practice four hours a day and play anything I wanted to on the violin (barring a decent up bow staccato that I'd never been able to do before), but I was still waiting for the other shoe to drop. Playing at home on my own terms was one thing, but could I survive in the real world of orchestra work? Even in a city as big as Toronto the musical community is small, and I didn't want to find out the hard way in a professional setting that I couldn't make the grade. Instead, I joined an amateur orchestra that was tackling a strenuous program. I passed with flying colors, handling all the demands of rehearsing and performing without any trouble. Finally, I knew that I'd made it. I started to play professionally again.

Working Again (Fall 1987)

Getting back to playing the violin was one thing; getting back to making a living was another. During the five years that I had been off work with my injury the music world in Toronto had changed significantly. Any limited connections I had were gone, whatever reputation I had begun to establish was forgotten, and employment-wise I was back at the proverbial square one. During my first season back at work, just one year after starting treatment with Barbara, I had the opportunity to do some wonderful things but I was a long way from full-time employment. My calendar was reminiscent of scenes of the Arctic tundra, with lots of very white, blank pages. But although I wasn't working a lot, I maintained a consistent practice schedule and felt that I was a stronger and better violinist than I had been before my injury. I finally believed in my health and my playing again, and at last stopped waiting for the other shoe to drop. Wrong again!

Second Season (Fall 1988)

By this time my calendar had started to fill in again. The fall of that year was extremely busy, with a three-week stretch of double and triple service days. Freelancing is usually a case of "feast or famine" and I hadn't faced this kind of workload since 1983. I knew I was doing a lot, but I was 100 percent recovered and felt that there was no reason to doubt that I could handle anything.

I was onstage during the last concert of this hectic three-week period when I felt that all-too-familiar twinge in my right arm. My immediate reaction was one of total and absolute disbelief – I must have been imagining it. A few moments later it happened again and the pain worsened until I couldn't deny it or ignore it. My arm felt exactly like it had so many times before, and I thought over two years of hard-won progress were slipping away over the course of a single symphony. I felt sick with the realization that the whole nightmare was starting over. As I struggled to make it to the end of the concert I felt that I was reliving my entire injury history, this time in fast-forward. The other shoe had dropped in a big way, long after I had stopped waiting for disaster. By the time the symphony ended I was in a lot of pain, I had trouble moving my arm and I was emotionally devastated.

Uppermost in my mind was fear of the worst-case scenario – that I would never be able to play. Maybe I just wasn't meant to be able to handle the demands of full-time playing. The best-case scenario I could envisage was another long and painful struggle back to health, although this time around I knew that with Barbara I would get the help I needed right away. As I waited for my appointment with her the next morning I was concerned not only about my shoulder, but also about how Barbara would react. In the past, medical professionals had put the blame on me when things had gone wrong. I had been following Barbara's advice to the letter and had tried to take her teaching and apply it to my work. Two years previously, it had been so important that Barbara believed in me. Now it was vitally important to me that Barbara know that I hadn't let her down. Her concern for my well-being was so genuine that if I were not able to play, it would be as much of a defeat for her as it was for me.

"Happily Ever After" . . . At Last!

All my fears were unfounded and this last setback didn't result in any of the awful things I had envisaged. Instead, it turned out to be the key to solving the mystery of what had happened seven years before. It gave Barbara and me the missing part of the puzzle and we were able to learn how my shoulder problem could be prevented. This relapse was an accelerated recreation of what had happened back in 1983, but this time around treatment consisted of just five sessions with Barbara. By taking prompt action and getting the correct diagnoses and treatment right off the bat, I didn't have to miss five years, five months, or even five days of playing. I haven't missed a day of work because of any playing injury problems since that time. Time off for a freelance musician is a precious commodity, and I fully intend to use all of mine for sensible pursuits like Caribbean vacations.

Thanks to Dr. X, I will always be more susceptible to shoulder problems than someone who hasn't had their shoulder surgically "cleaned up." Thanks to my genes, I also have an extremely long neck that leaves me wide open to neck.

problems if I'm not careful. The fact that I'm a freelance player also means that I must cope with a schedule that often borders on the ridiculous. Despite all of this, I am able to play comfortably, without any limitations. I will never accept pain and discomfort as part and parcel of the package of music-making – and neither should you!

Chapter 4

An Introduction to Physiotherapy

Physiotherapy, like medicine, is both a science and an art. In Canada the science is taught during four years of university education in a faculty of medicine and is based upon knowledge derived from years of scientific medical research. Physiotherapists emerge with a Bachelor of Science in physiotherapy, then continue their scientific studies with endless postgraduate courses in order to keep up with ongoing research and professional protocols.

The Art of Physiotherapy is simply the ability to make that science useful to patients and clients. These skills are first taught during internships in hospitals. As with all skills, they are improved and fine-tuned with countless hours of clinical practice.

After a time in general practice, usually in a hospital, many physiotherapists develop a special interest in one clinical area. This could be, for instance, neurology, cardio-respirology, rheumatology, gerontology, pediatrics, or my own preference, orthopedics. This decision to specialize engenders pursuit of every available postgraduate course in that subject and an ever increasing library of recommended journals and textbooks. As one's scientific knowledge increases and the art develops, patients generally respond more quickly and the pleasure of practicing physiotherapy is such that one cannot ever imagine doing anything else. Perhaps we resemble musicians.

Orthopedic physiotherapy is best described as a detective game. The physiotherapist plays the part of Sherlock Holmes and the patient is the client. The injury is the crime. The patient's story is the anecdotal evidence and provides the first clues. Evidence is gathered by a systematic examination of every relevant posture and movement and the joints involved. Then all the so-called "soft tissues" are tested, meaning ligaments, muscles, tendons, reflexes and sensation, or normal feeling. Close attention is paid to what the client wants to be able to do and which body postures and movements are necessary to perform these tasks.

This meticulous examination, although time-consuming, is also a necessary safety factor for patients. One needs to be certain that the patient's pain is not due to some underlying medical condition, as some internal organs can refer pain to other parts of the body, mimicking muscle and joint pains. Any suspicion that this is the case means a quick referral to a medical doctor for consultation. Physicians and physiotherapists work closely together and speak the same language of orthodox medicine.

Spinal x-rays are seldom necessary unless the patient's story includes a fall or some trauma that could have caused a cracked bone. X-rays only show bones and these are very seldom the cause of neck or back pain. Also, normal spinal x-ray reports can frighten people quite unnecessarily when misunderstood. Everyone over the age of thirty will show signs of normal wear and tear unless they are habitual couch potatoes. The way a qualified radiologist describes these normal signs of the aging process can terrify the subject of the x-rays unless it is quickly explained that they are simply showing the patient's age and amount of activity.

Finally, the detective-physiotherapist analyzes all of this information, makes a diagnosis and suggests a solution. For treatment to be successful, there must be close cooperation between the physiotherapist and the client/patient. Neither can achieve much in isolation, but together they make a very effective team.

Physiotherapists' tasks are complex. First they must diagnose the problems, then explain them very clearly to their patients, teaching all necessary anatomy and physiology in laymen's language. Next, providing patients agree to whatever treatment is suggested, the physiotherapists treat the injuries. Finally the most important part of any physiotherapy treatment is ensuring that patients are able to perform their job or any task or sport they wish to do, without immediately running into trouble with injuries again. This is where teamwork between physiotherapists and patients really pays off. The patients become the tutors and describe in detail, with practical demonstrations, precisely what, where and how they function. The physiotherapists then explain how these thing can be done without hurting the body and without compromising the patients' skills. This interesting exercise is called "ergonomics."

Once patients are painfree, have mastered any injury-prevention exercises deemed necessary and have corrected their ergonomics, there is no further need of physiotherapy intervention. Most soft tissue injuries recover within a six- to eight-week period as the body has amazing recuperative and healing abilities when it is not repeatedly abused.

Informed patients can usually self-monitor and self-manage any previously injured areas of their bodies and should not have to depend upon regular repetitive treatment of any description. If my patients keep returning, I know I have either been ineffective or have misdiagnosed the problem and must start again.

Although patients of all ages come to my clinic seeking help for every conceivable ache, pain or injury, there are among them four major groups. These are injured workers, injured athletes, motor vehicle accident victims and hurt children. Each group has different needs and requires a different approach to gain successful rehabilitation and return to their normal lifestyles.

When Christine Harrison arrived and stated that she was a violinist, unable to work because of an injury, I mentally placed her in the "injured workers" category. However, as I listened to her long, sad history and examined her acutely painful shoulder, it soon became evident that this was an incorrect assumption. Despite all that she had suffered and despite years of trying and failing, when I asked for her long-term and short-term goals, she said she just wanted to play her violin.

This is precisely the response one gets from injured athletes. If a dedicated runner falls and injures a leg, he will generally accept treatment of any kind, or even undergo surgery without complaint, as long as there is a chance that he will be able to run again. During the rehabilitation stage of recovery he will punish his body mercilessly in the gymnasium and do far too many repetitions of every prescribed exercise unless his physiotherapist and coach closely monitor his activity. If he thinks he is not recovering fast enough, he may start reaching out for alternatives to medicine and add naturopathy, acupuncture, chiropractic, massage, reflexology and many others to his regime. *Anyone* who will promise to speed his return to running is guaranteed this athlete's full attention and compliance–no matter how strange the advice or treatment.

"Normal," average, working people would settle for a sitting occupation for a while and slowly nurse their injured limb back to normal function with a few exercises each day. Athletes are not like this. They desperately miss their particular sport, and pursue regaining the ability to perform it with almost fanatical determination. They are wonderful patients and a joy to teach.

Christine belonged to the elite athlete group. I had discovered the Athletic Musician.

With appropriate orthopedic physiotherapy treatment and a carefully paced return to playing, Christine did recover full function. It was the realization that she need never have sustained her injuries or endured five years of pain and frustration that prompted the two of us to start teaching an injury-prevention-physiotherapy workshop called "Playing Without Pain." The response was so immediate and the need so apparent that I opened the Stouffville Musicians' Physiotherapy Clinic where we could teach and treat injured musicians. Christine became the Clinic's consultant for string musicians.

Orthopedic physiotherapists are generally very conservative clinicians and therefore are *safe to consult*. We view surgery as a last resort, rather than a "quick fix," and prefer ice packs rather than medication for the relief of pain from simple strains and sprains. Athletes have always treated soft tissue injuries thus. Although qualified to manipulate, we seldom see the need to do this, as we can usually gain good results with less passive methods within the patient's control. We have no patience with "press and guess" diagnostics, or the "fake and bake" approach to treatment of injuries. Much of our time has to be spent debunking myths, superstition and totally unscientific beliefs about injuries and treatments before we can teach self-help and self-care to musicians. "Old husbands' tales" abound, as everyone you meet has an opinion on injury prevention and health.

Orthopedic physiotherapists will never be satisfied until you can play without pain and will refer you to whoever else can help you the best if you do not show rapid objective signs of improvement in their care. For instance, I refer to the physiotherapist and occupational therapist in the Hand Clinic of our local hospital if hand trauma is the problem. They have far more specialized knowledge in this area than I.

I could listen to Christine play all day (which she must never do) and trust she will never need me, or anyone else, to treat her again.

PART II

Anatomy and
Applied Anatomy
for Musicians

Chapter 5

Anatomy for Musicians: or everything you wanted to know about necks, backs, shoulders, arms, and hands but were afraid to ask

Anatomy is not a dull subject. How we are constructed and how our bodies work is information that interests people of all ages, providing the facts are not made unintelligible by the use of obscure anatomical or medical language and terminology.

The Spine

The spine consists of many small bones (vertebrae) lined up one on top of another, with the skull at the top and the tail bone at the bottom (see fig. 1, p. 28) The neck consists of seven bones and the next twelve bones form the thorax or chest region and have the ribs attached to them. The next five bones form the low back or lumbar area. Below the low back, the next five bones have joined to make a solid piece called the sacrum, to which are attached the big pelvic bones you can feel above your hip joints. The small tail bones are attached to the bottom of the sacrum. Each bone (or vertebra) is shaped as in figure 2 (p. 29) with slight variations in different areas to allow special movements to occur, such as turning the head to look over the shoulder. Each vertebra has a body, which takes our weight in the upright position. Behind the body is a large hole, the vertebral foramen.

The bones are individually very strong and will seldom give trouble unless subjected to severe trauma or serious diseases. To break a small vertebra requires forces generated, for example, by diving into a pool with little or no water in it, or driving at high speed into a brick wall. The bony protuberances poking out from around the holes are not there for tweaking or tuning like an instrument, but for the attachment of ligaments holding the bones together and the many muscles needed to stabilize, protect and move the spine about.

Two little protuberances on each side join with those of the spinal bones

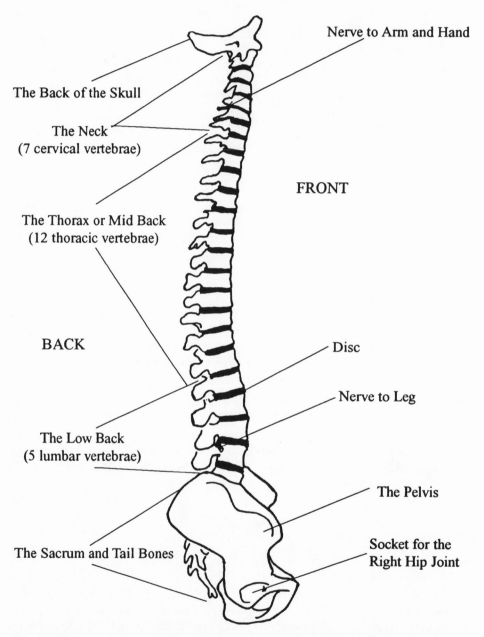

Nerve to Arm and Hand

The Back of the Skull

The Neck
(7 cervical vertebrae)

FRONT

The Thorax or Mid Back
(12 thoracic vertebrae)

BACK

Disc

Nerve to Leg

The Low Back
(5 lumbar vertebrae)

The Pelvis

The Sacrum and Tail Bones

Socket for the
Right Hip Joint

Fig. 1. The spine. This shows the vertebrae or bones of the spine and the discs, or shock absorbers, between them. The nerves emerge from behind the discs at every level.

FRONT

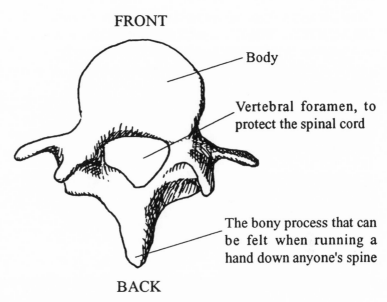

Body

Vertebral foramen, to
protect the spinal cord

The bony process that can
be felt when running a
hand down anyone's spine

BACK

Fig. 2. A vertebra viewed from above.

directly above and below, to form tiny joints called zygopophyseal joints. For
obvious reasons these are commonly called facet joints. They are very
tough,durable little joints designed to guide and limit the amount of movement
anatomically desirable between vertebrae. They seldom cause pain or problems,
even in extreme old age when they often appear grossly deformed or beaten-up
on x-ray examinations. Some people become quite addicted to "popping" these
facet joints by rapidly or forcefully rotating and twisting their necks or backs –
just as some like to "pop" their finger joints. Considering that the worst spinal
injuries include a history of twisting trauma, it is probably not a habit to be
recommended.

Nerves

With the spine assembled, the holes behind the bodies of the bones line up
to form a tube called the spinal canal. The top of this tube in the neck is directly
below a large hole in the bottom of the skull. Through this hole comes a thick
cord of nerves, the "spinal cord" which is protected by the spinal bones as it
passes down through their vertebral canal holes until it reaches the level of the
low back (see fig. 1, p. 28). At every space between the spinal bones, the cord
sends off a pair of nerves to parts of the body, one to the left side and one to the
right. These nerves are not imaginary or wispy, but are about the size of cooked

spaghetti. You can feel one on the inner side of the elbow where it passes through the groove designed to protect it on its way to the fourth and fifth fingers. Shortly after leaving the spinal canal, each nerve is covered with a protective outer sleeve, affording protection to the nerves as they pass through the body, like a house electric wiring system covered with insulation. Every nerve has a specific destination, supplying little nerve fibers to each muscle, tendon, ligament, joint, bone and area of skin, or dermatome, for which it is responsible (see fig. 3, p. 31). The nerves that leave the spine in the area of the neck travel down under the big neck muscles and across the top of the first rib in a thick bundle, down through the armpit and spread down the arm to the fingers, rather like a telephone system.

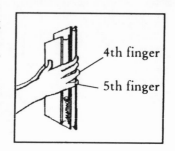

The nerves that leave the spine at the level of each vertebra in the thorax or mid-back travel around to the front of the body inside the muscles between each rib, giving off little nerve fibers to the ribs, muscles and skin as they pass, similar to a string vest. Nerves emerging from the low back region are going to supply the legs and feet. Several join together to cross the buttock and spread down the back of the leg. These are the largest, thickest nerves in the body and are called the sciatic nerves. They are about as thick as a finger as they cross diagonally downward from the spine and through the buttocks to reach the back of each thigh. The nerves then branch out again, descending through the leg to the feet and toes. Nerve pain down the back of the leg is called sciatica (see illus. 1, p. 32) and can spread as far as the heel or the big toe in severe cases. A separate nerve leaves the spine slightly higher up from the sciatic nerve and travels around to the front of the hip area, supplying the muscles and skin on the front of each thigh and knee.

This complex system of nerves is our body's communication system. Think of the brain as an intelligent computer. It sends orders and messages down the spinal cord and out to every area of the body via the nerves. Simultaneously, the nerves send back information about what is going on. Hence, when a musician wishes to play a tune, the brain sends the orders down the nerves to the fingers, telling them which muscles to use and how fast. The fingers, in turn, send back messages such as "I am too cold," "too stiff," "have not practiced enough," or "Eureka, how was that!?"

Discs

In between the bodies of each vertebra from the second down lies a very

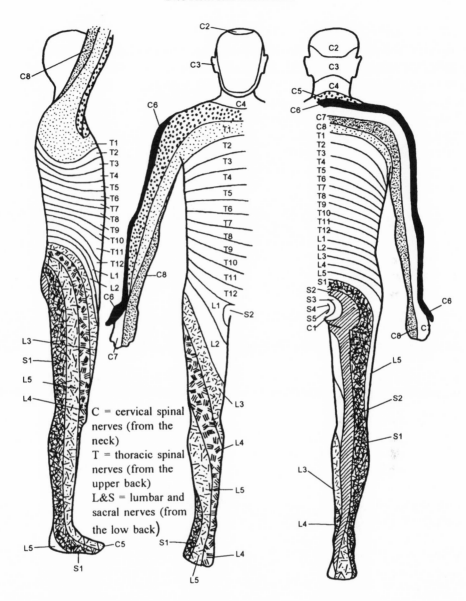

Fig. 3. Dermatomes. Dermatomes are the areas of the skin where feeling is supplied by the spinal nerves as they travel from the spine to every area of the body. The numbers indicate which part of the spine they come from.

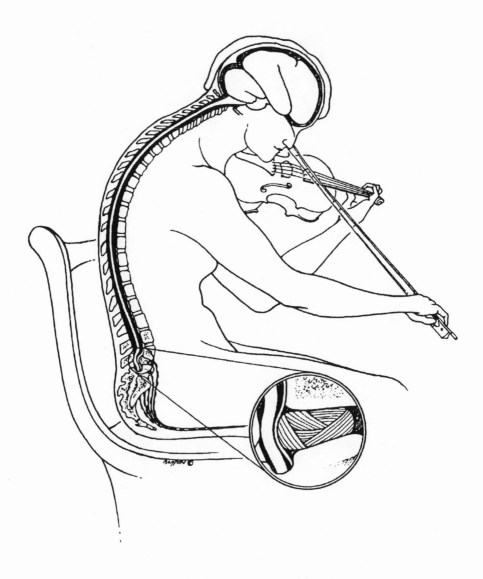

Illustration 1. Back and leg pain (sciatica) caused by prolonged, poor sitting posture.

Nucleus
This is like thick jelly, with a high water content, similar to gel toothpaste.

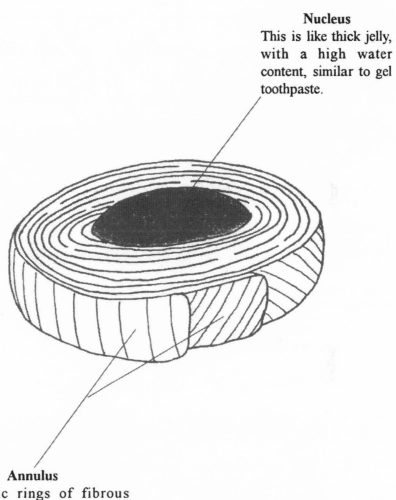

Annulus
Concentric rings of fibrous material surrounding the nucleus. The fibers of each layer run in different directions for added strength.

Fig. 4. The disc: Your spine's shock absorber.

important structure, the intervertebral disc. Discs are the same shape as the bodies of the vertebrae to which they are attached. They consist of almost continuous rings of fibrous material, layer upon layer, like an onion, with the fibers in each layer running at an angle to the next layer (see fig. 4, p. 33). The center or nucleus of the disc is roughly the consistency of gel toothpaste, with the fibrous layers (the annulus) surrounding this jelly. In a child or young person, the discs are very thick and strong with a high fluid content. They are very effective shock absorbers for running, jumping, sitting down hard and falling. Throughout life, discs can take a lot of weight if it is distributed evenly over their surfaces. Hence, in the upright position, people can carry heavy loads on their heads and shoulders or hips without being hurt. Each disc grows right into the body of the vertebra above and below it. Discs cannot be separated from the bones and it is absolutely impossible for them to "slip" out of place.

Unlike nerves and bones which are designed to last a lifetime, discs appear to have been designed as shock absorbers to get us safely through childhood and wild youth. Once we have reached our mid-twenties and are less likely to fall out of trees or high chairs, or take part in body-punishing sports, discs start to dry out, crack, and generally deteriorate (see fig. 5, p. 35). This process gradually continues through middle and old age and is the reason that old people are shorter than when they were young. Degenerating or deteriorating discs is not a disease and does not hurt. It happens to everyone on this planet. If you are over thirty years old and your spinal x-ray report shows narrowing spaces between several vertebrae, interpreted as "degenerating discs," that is a normal x-ray. The person examining you or x-raying you probably has exactly the same signs, unless they are very young and have avoided physical work.

Normal movements of the neck and back affect the intervertebral discs. When we bend our necks to look down or bend over to touch our toes, the front of the spinal bones move closer together to curve the neck or back forward. The discs between the bones are squeezed at the front and they behave just like jelly donuts. The jelly-like center slowly oozes through the disc, away from the squeeze and pushes against the strong, outer disc wall at the opposite side, causing a bulge at the back of each disc. When the squeeze is removed, the bulge slowly subsides and the jelly returns to the center (see fig. 6, p. 36).

There is room available for small, normal disc bulges. This is how discs behave and it does not hurt. Every time we look down to read or write, the neck discs will slowly start to bulge at the back. Whenever musicians hold their heads tilted to one side for a period of time, their neck discs will bulge on the opposite side. Bending over to fasten shoes causes the lower back discs to bulge at the back–and so does sitting in a relaxed, slouched position. When the back and neck return to an upright posture, the discs gradually return to their original shape. CT scans of people without back pain or neck pain frequently show these small bulges that normally occur with the movement of the spine.

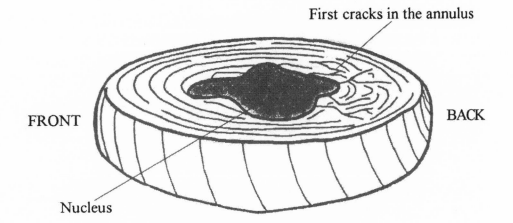

First cracks in the annulus

FRONT   BACK

Nucleus

Middle-Aged Disc: over 30 years of age

- Thinner
- Cracks appear, starting at the back, where the disc has bulged most often
- The disc is starting to "self-destruct"
- Disc degeneration is normal and does not hurt

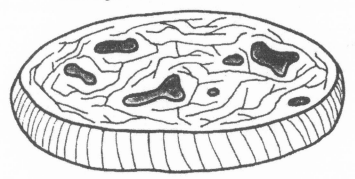

Old Disc: over 80 years of age

- Very thin. Very cracked. "Dried-out"
- Very little, if any, bulging of the disc occurs when we bend
- Annulus and nucleus no longer defined
- Old people are shorter and generally suffer less from backache and neck ache

Fig. 5. Disc degeneration.

Discs behave like jelly donuts when they are squeezed. Bending the neck or low back forward for a while causes young, healthy discs to bulge at the back. There is room for normal-sized bulges and they do not cause pain. When you straighten up, the bulges subside and the jelly returns to the middle.

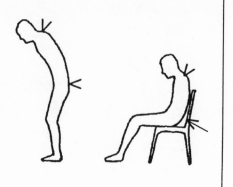

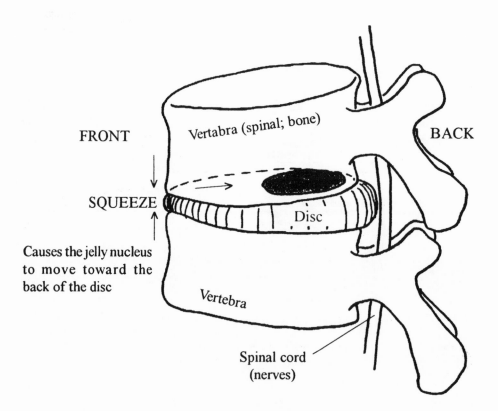

FRONT Vertabra (spinal; bone) BACK

SQUEEZE

Causes the jelly nucleus to move toward the back of the disc

Disc

Vertebra

Spinal cord (nerves)

Fig. 6. How discs behave when we bend.

It is interesting to note that the incidence of neck and back pain problems diminishes quite dramatically with age. Very few people seeking help are over fifty years old and those who still have a problem at age sixty usually have bodies that appear much younger. Backache and neckache, like good wine, improve with age.

As the same cannot truthfully be said for any other part of the body, one is forced to conclude that our discs are to blame for most common spinal problems. Yet their aging process is designed to be a painless procedure. What goes wrong?

The fault lies in our lifestyles and unnatural stresses we place upon the spine and discs, causing the outer fibrous rings of some of the discs to crack and fissure too soon in life. The first cracks in the outer fibrous layers can occur quite early in life if the spine is subjected to direct trauma or very heavy physical work, including bending to lift weights, or if it is held in an awkward position for long periods of time. These first cracks occur in the part of the disc that is bulged most often or most vigorously. Generally speaking, the positions most musicians overuse are poking the head forward, or bending the neck forward or sideways, or keeping it twisted. They also allow the low back to bend and sag by sitting slouched or bending over slightly to play (see photos 1, 2, 3, 4 and 5, pp. 38-42).

Children tolerate twisted neck positions better than adults only because the disc walls are strongest in childhood. Sustained or frequently repeated twisting movements also serve to hasten the formation of cracks in the fibrous outer layer of the discs involved, probably by weakening and separating the angled fibers, rather like untwisting a woven basket. When this happens, the squeezing that occurs during spinal bending movements and maintained bending positions causes the discs to bulge much further than they should, because the amount of jelly in them has not yet diminished with age. The space behind the disc is not sufficient to accommodate this larger bulge and it comes into contact with the spinal cord (nerves). If you apply pressure to spinal nerves, they produce pain—just like touching an exposed nerve in a tooth. Applying any pressure to the front of the spinal cord in the neck in this way causes an ache across the back of the neck and shoulders and down between the shoulder blades. These aches have a physical cause and are not due to stress or tense playing. In the low back it can cause an ache across the whole of the low back area, sometimes spreading into the buttocks (see illus. 2, p. 43).

If these aches are ignored, or simply treated by any method giving only momentary relief, the problems usually recur and gradually increase in severity over time. This is why massage, ice packs, manipulation, drugs, TENS machines, acupuncture, pressure point therapy, chiropractic "adjustments" and all the other therapies that have been invented for pain relief have to be repeated endlessly. None of them addresses the cause of the problem and an unhealthy life-long dependency often ensues. The affected discs continue to crack up and the amount

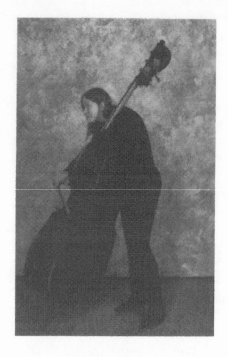

Poor playing posture. The head is held forward, in front of the body when looking upward. This position is frequently responsible for headaches, as it compresses the top neck joint.

Correct playing position

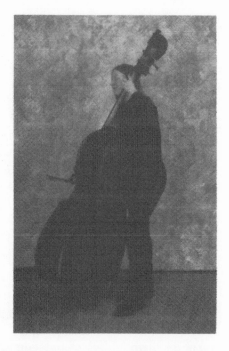

Photo 1. The bass player's posture.

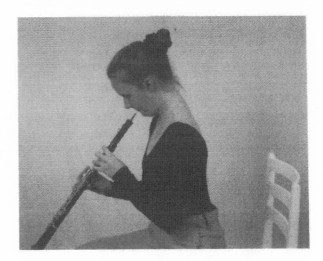

Poor neck posture

Correct posture

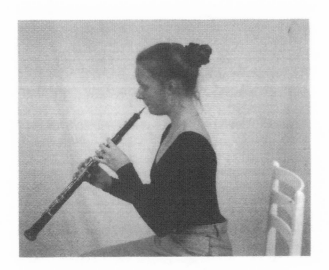

Photo 2. The oboist's posture.

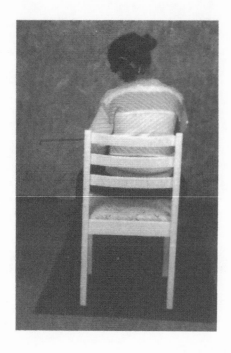

Poor playing posture. Cellist playing
with twisted neck.

Corrected playing position

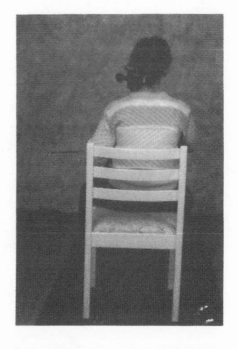

Photo 3. The cellist's posture.

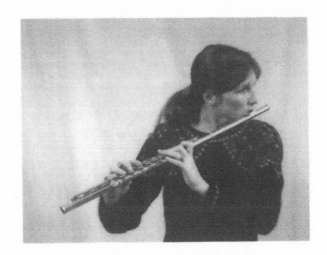

Poor playing posture with neck in a twisted playing position.

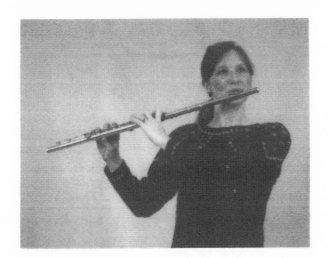

Corrected posture

Photo 4. The flautist's posture.

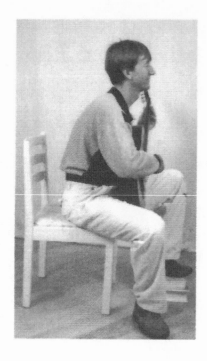

A poor playing posture for a guitarist with the head held forward from the body and the back slouched

A corrected playing posture assumes an erect position that feels awkward at first, but improves with practice

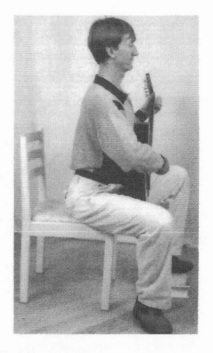

Photo 5. The guitarist's posture.

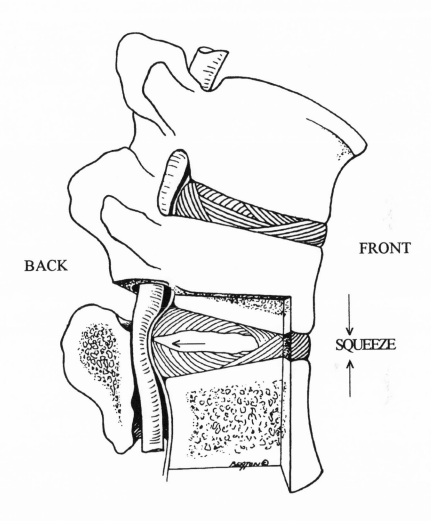

This illustration shows how a disc is affected by bending the spine forward too often or for too long. Note how the disc is bulging at the back and pressing aginst the spinal cord, causing pain.

Illustration 2. Common low backache.

of bulging steadily increases until the bulge is forced to squeeze around to the side of the spinal cord in its search for more space. This space is where the spinal nerves are leaving the spine on their journeys to the limbs or around the trunk. When the bulging disc comes into contact with one of these nerves, pain spreads down the nerve to wherever it goes. The more pressure exerted upon the nerve, the further away from the spine the pain spreads (see illus. 3, p. 45).

Nerve root fibers respond to pressure first by transmitting pain back to the brain, requesting help. If help is not forthcoming and the pressure continues, the nerves transmit more severe pain signals and eventually numbness in the area of the body they supply. The same nerves now can no longer transmit detailed messages from the brain to their muscles, so these muscles begin to lose strength and control. Hence, disc pressure on a nerve leaving the neck to supply the hand interferes significantly with the musician's ability to perform. If the pressure is removed and not reinflicted, the nerve recovers. If the disc finally splits, or herniates (see fig. 7, p. 46 and fig. 8, p. 47), the pain is constant, day and night, and may progress through numbness and muscle weakness before recovery occurs. The recovery may be instantaneous or take many weeks depending upon how much pressure has been applied to the nerve and for how long. Nerves to your hands and legs do recover from this kind of disc pressure eventually, without surgical intervention and with the right kind of help and advice.[1]

Discs cannot "slip" out of place, nor can they be "popped" back again. This is yet another old husbands' tale.

Lordosis

Animal spines are roughly the same design as human spines, but their discs are not subjected to the same squeezing forces because animals seldom have to bend forward–their spines stay horizontal and straight. Apart from eating and drinking, animals hold their necks straight, carrying their heads higher than their backs (see illus. 4, p. 48).

Humans, on the other hand, having adopted the upright position, are forced to bend forward to do most everyday activities, such as washing our face or brushing our teeth. Our spines do have some built-in protection however, which animals do not. These are curves in the spine which appear when we are old enough to hold up our head and to stand up. One curve is in the neck area and the other in the low back (see illus. 5, p. 49). Each curve is called a *lordosis*. Babies' spines tend to stay in a rounded or fetal position much of the time, but when they stand up a reverse curve or lordosis is easily identified in their necks and low backs.

A lordosis is nature's way of protecting the discs in both of these overworked areas. The curves pull the backs of the vertebrae closer together in both the neck

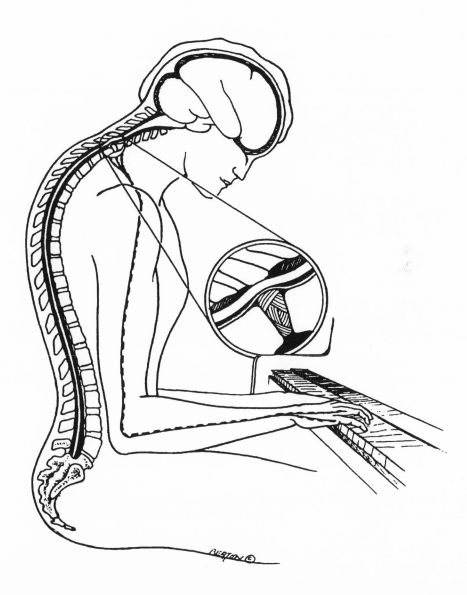

Illustration 3. Hand problems referred from the neck. Tingling and numbness in the fourth and fifth fingers caused by bending the neck forward for too long. This musician would probably complain of pain across the back of the shoulders and between the shoulder blades.

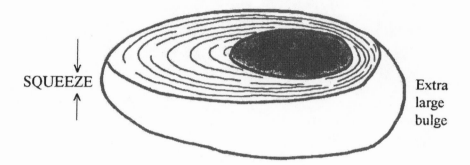

SQUEEZE

Extra
large
bulge

Discs do not slip. If they are squeezed too hard
or too often in the same direction, they will form
an extra large bulge.

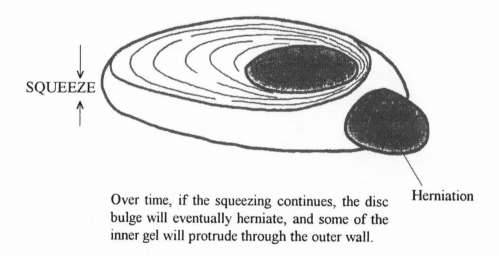

SQUEEZE

Herniation

Over time, if the squeezing continues, the disc
bulge will eventually herniate, and some of the
inner gel will protrude through the outer wall.

Fig. 7. "Slipped discs."

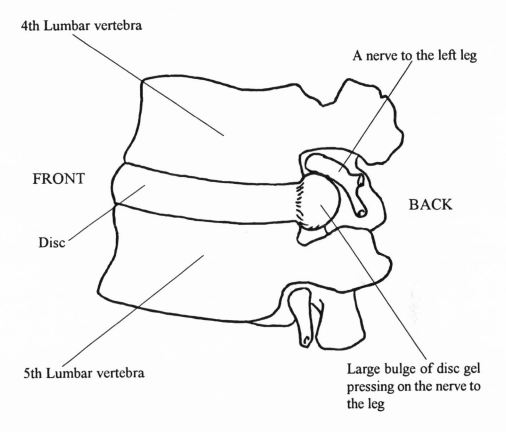

4th Lumbar vertebra

A nerve to the left leg

FRONT

BACK

Disc

5th Lumbar vertebra

Large bulge of disc gel pressing on the nerve to the leg

Fig. 8. A herniated disc causing sciatica.

Animals' spines are similar to our own, but they seldom have to bend forward. If curled up to sleep, they frequently stretch by arching backward before resuming activity.

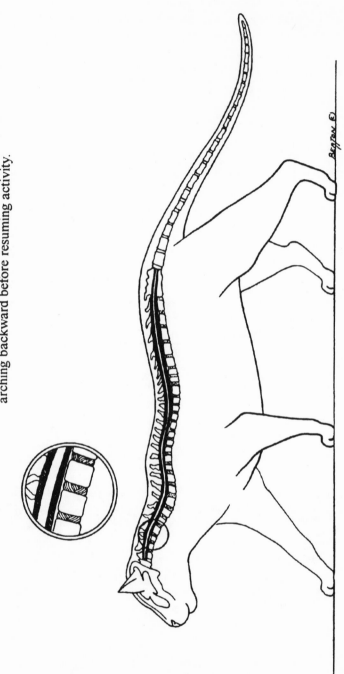

Illustration 4. The spine of a typical animal.

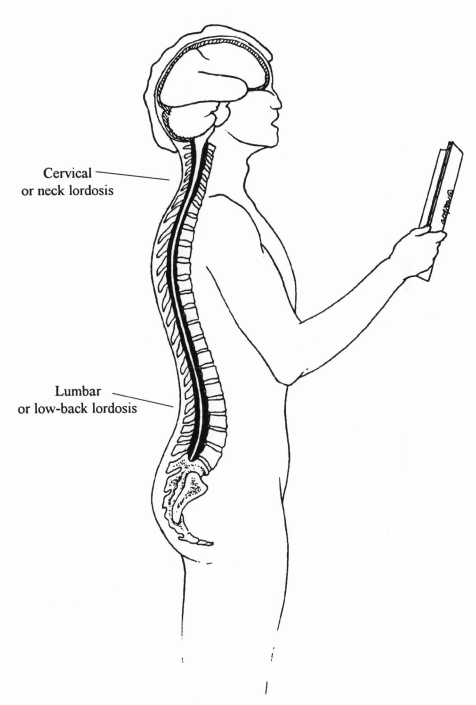

Cervical
or neck lordosis

Lumbar
or low-back lordosis

Illustration 5. Neck and low-back lordoses in a singer with excellent posture.

and the low-back, thus squeezing the backs of the discs between those bones. This pushes the jelly centers of the discs forward, away from the spinal cord and nerve roots and away from any of the cracks developing toward the back of the discs. Skaters landing hard on the ice after performing double or triple jumps invariably aim to land with their heads up and their backs arched for protection. Gymnasts jumping from high beams or rings try to land the same way. Professional weight lifters can press weights far heavier than average people would ever attempt, and come to no harm if they keep their heads up and maintain a lordosis in their low backs while lifting.

Throughout history, arches have been built to add strength to structures such as bridges and viaducts. Your back and neck's lordotic arches provide strength and stability for your spine when you work or perform. A normal lordosis is your back and neck's best friend.

Providing that your posture is upright and well balanced, with both lordoses evident, it is very difficult to hurt your neck or your back. So your grandmother was right–good posture is very important.

Note

1. Dr. J. Cyriax: *Textbook of Orthopaedic Medicine, Vol.1., Diagnosis of Soft Tissue Lesions.* Baillière & Tindall.

Chapter 6

Taking Care of Your Neck and Back

Standing Posture

Unfortunately, for the past thirty years, most medical practitioners in North America were taught to treat low back pain by flattening the low back curve or *lumbar lordosis*. It is difficult to understand how this thinking developed, as a flattened lordosis is one of the first signs of a painful back. Why would anyone wish to stay in that position unless forced to? This faulty philosophy slowly trickled down to physiotherapists, nurses, fitness experts and all others dealing with injuries or fitness.

Postural exercises included a movement to flatten the low back, called the "pelvic tilt" – a movement necessary for belly dancing and sexual intercourse, but resulting in a very odd standing posture. It is hard to imagine a skater being able to attempt a jump while maintaining a pelvic tilt position. A sprinter certainly could not sprint, and you would not be able to run to catch a bus. Hopefully the sustained pelvic tilt posture will soon die a natural death, because your lordosis is your back's best friend.

To stand with good posture, simply stand as tall as possible, relax the shoulder girdle and breathe normally. Examined from the side, your head should be balanced on your neck so that it is not jutting forward, ahead of your body. Lifting the chest bone (sternum) slightly helps you to stand erect with less effort, and there is no need to force the shoulders backward as in an exaggerated military posture. If you think your stomach is sticking out, pull it in, but do not tuck your hips under you to complete a pelvic tilt. Your knees should be straight, but not locked back, and your weight should be more toward the front of your feet than the back. Once balanced, very little muscle work is necessary to maintain the erect position and many vague neck and back aches are immediately eased.

Occasionally we see musicians who have developed a backward swaying posture which balances them in a very poor position. The upper body leans backward from the waist, and the head leans forward to counteract that weight. Most of the bodyweight goes through the heels and the rear of the feet. This posture will eventually lead to posturally induced pain in several areas of the neck and back. One simple maneuver that seems to help correct this posture is to place one foot on a block or stool in front. The neck posture will also need correcting (see photo 6, p. 53) as a swayback posture usually causes the head to poke forward, to maintain balance.

All musicians should develop and maintain excellent posture. Not only does your body appreciate it, but it helps to impart a sense of "presence" which accompanies successful artists (see photo 7, p. 54).

Good posture should not be static because your body likes to move frequently. Learn to walk and move gracefully, maintaining the same good standing posture demonstrated by singers, gymnasts, ballet dancers, matadors and the Queen. Sitting posture, the position most musicians are forced to use for performing, will be discussed in detail later in this chapter.

Taking Care of Your Neck and Back

Once spinal anatomy is understood, it is easier to appreciate that the most common neck and back problems are caused by the way we misuse our spines each day, rather than by obscure diseases or trauma. So many myths abound about what is "good" or "bad" for your neck or back. We will now address everyday activities which can affect the well-being of your body and will, hopefully, be able to correct any misinformation you have already collected.

Beds, Pillows, and Sleeping Posture

Let's start with your bed. Is it so comfortable that you love to get into it and feel rested and pain-free after a night's sleep? That is the only way to judge if you have the right bed for you. It can be hard, medium, soft, foam, futon, waterbed or nails. None have any outstanding merit, it simply depends on what size and shape you are. Most women have curved figures, so if they try to sleep on a firm bed they are miserable because nothing supports where they curve inward. Similarly, men with broad shoulders and narrow hips have to lie in a sideways curve when lying on their sides on a firm bed, just to reach the bed with their bodies. So a firm bed is not necessarily superior. Do not take anyone's advice about what type of bed is "right" for you, just sleep on as many different kinds of mattresses as you can, until you find the bed that feels just right. If this is difficult to accomplish, experiment with your own bed. Try sleeping on top of your comforter, then try sleeping on your mattress or a sleeping bag on the floor. You will soon discover what your body prefers. You should start each day feeling your best (unless, of course, the after-show party got out of hand – but that is another story).

Similarly, the best position to sleep in is any position you like. There is

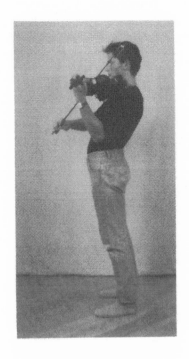

Swayback posture. A poor playing position, caused by leaning backward from the waist, and poking the head forward to maintain balance

The corrected swayback posture

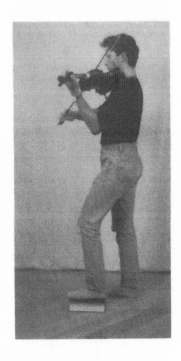

Photo 6. Swayback posture.

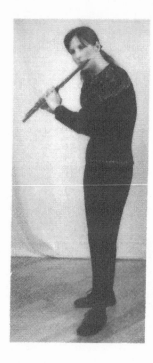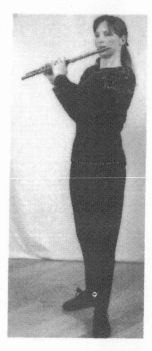

A poor playing posture (far left) and a good playing position (left)

An excellent neck and back posture in a sitting position

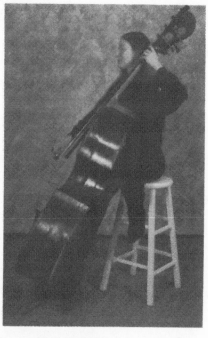

Photo 7. Good posture imparts a sense of presence.

nothing wrong with lying like a pretzel or sleeping on your stomach if you are comfortable, sleep well and awaken without any aches or pains. There really should be no need to put pillows between your knees or behind your back. Turning over in bed must be like Vesuvius erupting when all these extra props have to turn. If you are in pain, however, use anything that allows you to rest comfortably.

Pediatricians inform us that newborn babies should not be placed on their stomachs to sleep, but their advice does not extend to young people and adults. Most people find that their necks object to being twisted all night, so stomach sleepers in the prone position are advised to pull up one knee and turn slightly toward that side, to take the twist off their neck discs (see fig. 9, p. 56).

The fetal position is probably the worst for everyone over the age of one. Just think of the backward forces it exerts upon your discs all night.

Pillows

Pillows should support the neck rather than the head. One should be sufficient, and feathers are still the best filling. Feather pillows can be tucked and pushed into any position to support your particular design and length of neck, and they will remain that shape, rather than bouncing back to a preformed foam shape. Search for a feather-proof cover if you suffer from allergies. If you use several pillows to prop up your head, the jelly in your neck discs will be squeezed backward or sideways, bulging toward the spinal cord and nerves all night and you can awaken with arm, hand and neck aching, tingling or numbness symptoms. This can also happen if you take a large pillow into a waterbed. If your body weight displaces water toward the edges of the bed, the added height plus a pillow can push your head and neck into too much forward or sideways bending. Try a much smaller pillow in the curve of your neck when you lie on your back. If you have very broad shoulders you may need two pillows or one doubled over when you sleep on your side. Otherwise, your neck may be bent sideways all night.

If you like to read or watch television in bed, lie on your side or stomach. Never lie on your back and prop up your head and shoulders. Think of your discs' anatomy and you will understand why this position can get you into trouble (as previously pointed out). Considering that we spend roughly one-third of our lives in bed, it makes sense to spend time ensuring that those hours help us to recover from the physical stresses of the rest of the day, rather than adding to them.

Eventually Everyone Has to Get Out of Bed

During the hours spent sleeping or resting, spinal discs draw in fluid and nutrition from their adjacent vertebrae. Hence, when you first get up, you are

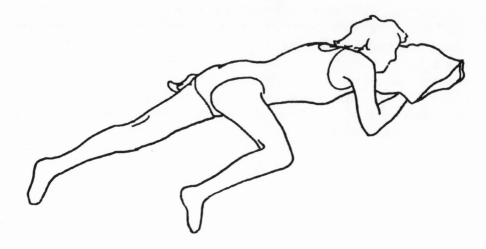

Fig. 9. Comfortable sleeping position for many people.

taller than at other times of the day and your discs can bulge further and more easily when you bend. Once upright, gravity and the weight of your head and body press down on each disc and they gradually lose their extra height and fluid content. (This accounts for having to alter the position of your car rearview mirror at the end of your day.) It is not a good idea, therefore, to stress your spine when you first get out of bed, as normal, small disc bulges can be made much larger then. Weight lifters do not usually do heavy lifting practice early in their day, so consider putting out heavy garbage before you go to bed. Help your children to climb safely to wherever you want them, rather than picking them up to speed up the family's early morning rush hour.

Similarly, early morning exercises should not include touching your toes or doing sit-ups. Instead, do yawning and backward stretching. Taking an early morning walk or jog is beneficial; sitting slumped at the breakfast table obviously is not.

Sitting Posture and Chairs

Sitting stresses your back. Several years ago, a renowned Swedish orthopedist, Professor Alf Nachemson, conducted a series of scientific experiments to measure which postures stressed discs in the low back, and how severely. His subjects were healthy young students and his results have influenced injury prevention programs in industry and sport throughout the world. One part of his research demonstrated that both the sitting position and standing while bent forward exert approximately 50 percent more stress on the low back discs than standing up straight. Therefore, people who sit for many hours each day or habitually bend forward to work are stressing their low backs far more than those who stand or walk about. For musicians, the majority of whom sit to play, my advice is to sit as little as possible at all other times.

Children instinctively do just about everything right until they've been trained to do otherwise. Children seldom sit. Trying to persuade them to sit still during a prolonged car or bus ride used to be well nigh impossible as they fidgeted due to increasing discomfort. Fortunately, seat belt legislation came to the aid of cross parents and drivers, and children are now tied into their seats with "straight-jacket" harnesses that don't give them room to stand or lie down even if they go to sleep. This is obviously preferable to having them hurtle through the windshield in an accident, but I hope someone is still working on this problem of enforced sitting for safety.

Children, generally speaking, are either running around being very active, or lying about to read, watch TV or rest, ready for the next bout of high activity. They can hardly sit still long enough to eat. Gradually, with constant coaching at home and school, children are trained to sit. They still instinctively do things to help their backs and necks recover from the periods of enforced sitting, however. They lie on the floor a lot, usually on their stomachs, to read or do homework or watch TV. Often they will pull a pillow under their upper body to take some weight from their elbows, but allow their backs to remain curved backward.

This is a very effective recovery position for a spine that has worked hard or sat too long. Unfortunately, as soon as growing teenagers start to take up a lot of room on the floor, they're often told to sit on a chair to do their homework, etc., "like a normal human being" and many have special desk and chair sets bought by kindly relatives to get them up from underfoot. Hence, many adults gradually lose their ability to lie and rest or read in this position, and their bodies are denied a regular dose of recuperation from stressful postures (see fig. 10, p. 58).

When trapped into sitting, young people soon learn how to ease their backs and necks. They lean back to listen and lean forward to work (see photo 8, p. 59). They rest the weight of their heads on their hands and elbows on the dinner-table to survive a lengthy meal.

These are all very effective ways to ease your neck and low back, and get young people into trouble with parents and teachers every day. The children, however, are right. When one sits as recommended by many experts, with one's hips and knees at 90 degrees, and one's back firmly supported by an upright chair back, the experts may be happy but one's body is not. It is virtually impossible to maintain a lordosis in the low back to protect the discs in this position. Also, hip joints object. The position of comfort for a hip joint is at about 145 degrees, roughly the position adopted by horseback riders (see fig. 11, p. 60).

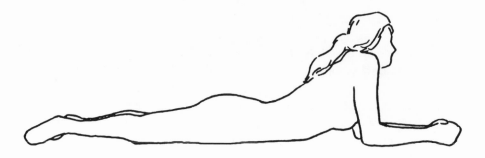

Fig. 10. Good recovery position for resting your back.

This position allows the spine to maintain its normal curves and also opens up the area at the front of the hip joints, where the main blood vessels enter and leave the leg. Thus, when young people tip their chairs forward, they're trying to maintain their low-back lordosis and when they tip their chairs backward or forward, they're easing their hip joints and increasing the circulation to and from their legs. When schools cunningly foiled the chair-tippers by switching to one-size-fits-all torture chairs with built-in writing tables, students could still slide their buttocks forward on the seats to increase the blood flow to their legs, but their low backs now sagged and ached, and they were unable to tip forward or perch on the front of the fixed chair to form a lordosis and alleviate the ache.

What can musicians learn from all of this? Obviously, to sit as seldom as possible! Do as children like to do – walk more, move more and lie about to rest and read. Stand to play whenever possible and keep moving. Take your weight from one foot to the other. Walk about while thinking, or lie down. There's nothing new about this – in 200 B.C. ancient Romans lay about on couches to survive their long feasts or just talk to each other.

It's always interesting to note that when companies request investigation of the reasons for numerous backache complaints among their workers, the majority of sufferers are sitting in offices or are salespeople sitting in cars all day.

Musicians, too, must sit or drive frequently for hours at a time. How you sit and what you sit upon are therefore of great importance if you are to avoid postural backache.

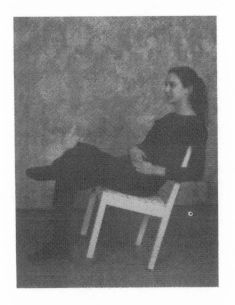

Teenager leans backward to ease her low back from the strain of sitting. This is a sensible thing to do.

Teenager tips and angles her book, to restore neck and low-back lordoses. This is also a good thing to do.

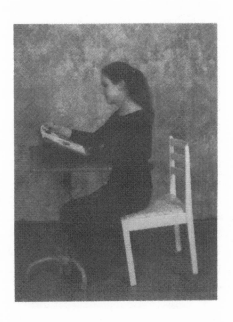

Photo. 8. How a young person copes with sitting.

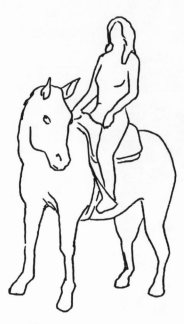

Fig. 11. Rider's posture.

Chairs

Chairs can be generally divided into three categories: 1) those which are carefully designed to keep the sitter comfortable and happy for hours (e.g., bar stools, top of the line car seats, some first-class airline seats, executives' adjustable chairs); 2) those which confine and control you for a specified length of time (all other airline seats, most car seats, theater seats, most children's seats); or 3) those designed for stacking, storage and ease of moving, for the benefit of caretakers, cleaners and stage hands, rather than the sitters.

When you have the power to choose, pick these correct ergonomic ingredients from the first group:

- Your knees should be lower than your hips, so sit on a high stool, or chair with a cushion. Ideally the seat height should be higher than your kneecaps when you stand beside the chair.

- Choose a seat or cushion which is higher at the back than the front. This will tilt your pelvis so that you can sit with a natural lordosis with very little effort. The amount of tilt is a personal preference and depends upon how flexible your spine is and how deep a lordosis you have. A wedge cushion can make all the difference, so experiment with the degree of tilt until you find what suits your back the best (see photo 9, p. 61). Some musicians have learned to put blocks under the back legs of their chairs.

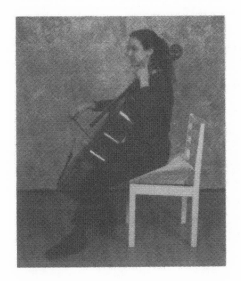

Photo 9. Using a wedge cushion to improve sitting position.

Photo 10. A good sitting posture with kneeling chair.

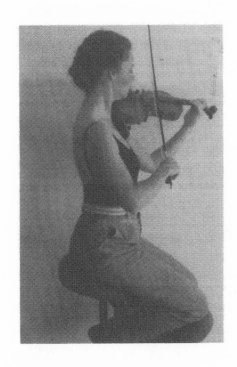

- The back of the chair isn't all that important. You may use it to lean against occasionally, for a rest from the upright position, but most sitting workers do not sit back to work and ache less quickly if they sit forward on the seats and stay erect.

- Executive chairs that allow you to lean back in the lazyboy position to rest or telephone are a great luxury for home or office – but are hardly practical for playing.

Avoid molded seats which are contoured as you are. It's very difficult to move about on seats like this and to survive sitting one should be able to shift and fidget easily. This is similarly the problem with fixed chair backs and supports which press into the low back region. These give short-term comfort by pushing into the lordosis, but backache is almost inevitable for young people having to sit too still, even with good support. (It's similar to backaches generated by mall-walking, when the same part of every joint takes the same weight with every step because the walking surface is so flat, hard and consistent.)

There should be sufficient padding on the seat to prevent your seat bones from pressing hard onto an unyielding surface. If you have built-in body padding, hard seats won't bother you as much, but bony individuals should cushion their seat bones. Again, the padding material must not prevent you from moving a little, often and easily. The front edge of the seat should be rounded or a waterfall design, to avoid pressure on the back of your thighs and the nerves to your lower legs and feet. The best design for a general working chair is still the kneeling-chair (see photo 10, p. 61). This combines the forward tilted seat with a shin rest which helps to take weight from the spine. It improves circulation to the legs and most knees don't mind this position at all. As when breaking in a new saddle, it's best to use this chair for gradually increasing periods of time, to allow your shins to become accustomed to taking weight. And remember not to lean back! Unfortunately for musicians, this design is more acceptable in front of a computer than a conductor.

The Wenger Corporation's Cello Chair was a vast improvement compared with most chairs musicians have to accept. The seat was higher (although not high enough for the majority of musicians) and tilted forward (although still tilted insufficiently). They were certainly on the right track. There will never be one chair which will please or suit all musicians, for obvious reasons, but Christine and I have recently designed a chair for Wenger which incorporates the basic essentials we think will be appreciated by most of you.

The seat is higher than the kneecaps of average height people. The front of the seat is "waterfalled" and the rear of the seat is a horizontal pad or perch for brief rests. When playing (or singing) the artist moves to the front of the seat and takes about one-third of the bodyweight through legs and feet. Already you can hear the groans from those musicians who have no strength or conditioning in their legs and prefer to sag onto a chair like a sack of potatoes!

While testing prototypes of this chair in the Clinic and during our various workshops, we found that musicians coping with injuries liked it at once. Singers loved it. Patients with industrial or sports injuries to their necks, shoulders or low backs preferred to sit on this chair for treatment sessions in the Clinic. All that remains to be done is to persuade healthy musicians to try this ergonomically designed playing chair and learn how to use it as a strong dose of injury-prevention medicine. Be warned that it is almost impossible to use a chair with a tilted seat while wearing slippery clothing. You will slowly slide off (see photo 11, p. 64). *When you have no choice* and must sit for a long time on poorly designed chairs from the second and third groups, there are many things you can do to survive while playing. Christine will address this in Chapter 9.

Driving and Car Seats

When driving is a large part of your life, buy the best seat and accept the car that goes with it. Avoid bucket seats like the plague. Your car seat, too, should slope forward, not backward. Correct a bucket seat by filling up the back half of the seat with a firm folded blanket to make the seat at least level. In small cars this can be a problem for tall people with little headroom (see fig. 12, p. 63).

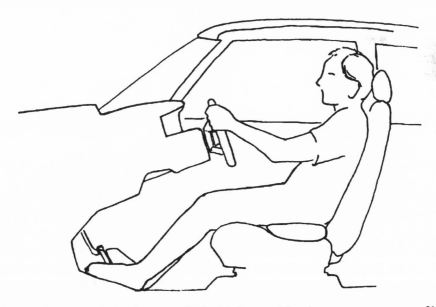

Fig. 12. Sports car's bucket seat. This driving position is a common cause of low backache. Fill in the bucket shape until the seat is horizontal providing an improved driving position.

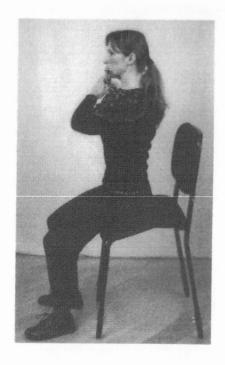

Good playing posture on Wenger Corporation's prototype Stouffville chair

Resting posture on Wenger Corporation's prototype Stouffville chair

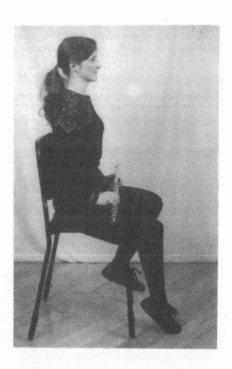

Photo 11. Wenger Corporation's prototype Stouffville chair.

A roll or small firm cushion in the small of your back will maintain your lordosis. Have several of different thickness, and interchange them on a long drive to vary the position for your back. When you're driving, keep the back of your seat upright to avoid having to hold your head poked forward to see as this position is very hard on the neck. Your headrest should be behind your head, not your neck. Whenever you remember to, pull your head back to touch the headrest briefly, keeping your eyes on the road and making a double chin. This counteracts the tendency to hold your head too far forward when driving. Another good habit, whenever you park or have come to a halt in traffic, is to put your head back and briefly examine the inside roof of your car.

On long journeys, leave time for a stop at least every hour – more often if you suffer from neckache or backache. Rather than sitting in the coffee shop, walk about a little and do the back bends prescribed in Chapter 10. If you are a passenger, recline your seat backward and put a roll behind your neck and your back to support your lordoses. Alter the reclining angle of the seat back every half hour to change the areas bearing weight in your spine.

The only good thing that can be said about sitting is that it becomes less of a problem with age. Once your discs have dried out a lot and degenerated a bit, you will find that you can sit comfortably for hours. Even then, a rocking chair is appreciated by very old joints, because rocking movements ease arthritic aches and your body always prefers a little movement rather than immobility.

Older people frequently forget the back and neck pains they suffered in their own youth. Please think of these things if you're teaching young children and adolescents to play, and encourage them to practice standing up. Theory can be discussed just as easily lying on the floor, propped up on your elbows, if you have not stiffened up too much to get into this position (see fig. 10, p. 58).

Lifting

Incorrect lifting techniques are responsible for many neck and back injuries. The trouble seems to stem from the fact that few people lift carefully unless the weight is excessive. In practice, most people are hurt by frequently and carelessly lifting quite small weights, such as groceries, small children, speakers and instrument cases (see illus. 6, p. 66).

The low back is safe when it is held rigidly in its curved lordosis to lift. Lifting is done by bending the hips or the knees or both but never the spine (see fig. 13, p. 67). The worst lifting injuries I have seen have involved more than one person doing the lift, or have incorporated a twisting movement of the back. Examples are snow shoveling and twisting to throw the snow to one side, or running after a ball, bending to pick it up and then twisting quickly to throw it. Two-person lifts are fine if they are coordinated, but if one partner suddenly

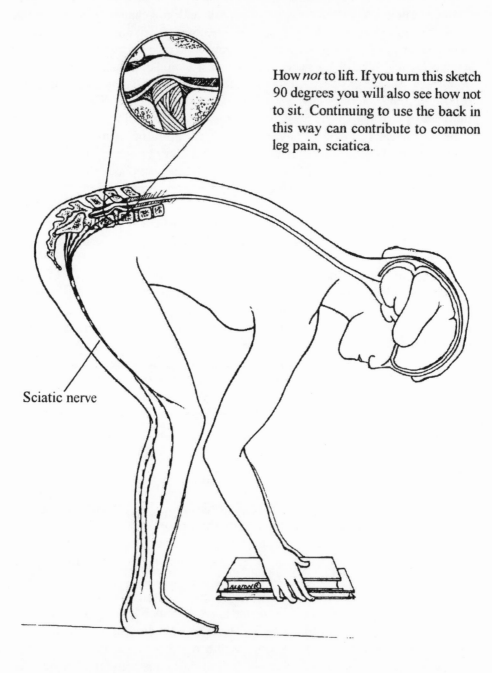

How *not* to lift. If you turn this sketch 90 degrees you will also see how not to sit. Continuing to use the back in this way can contribute to common leg pain, sciatica.

Sciatic nerve

Illustration 6. Back pain and sciatica caused by incorrect lifting or prolonged sitting with knees higher than hips.

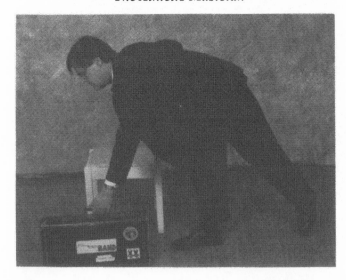

Photo 12. The "golfer's lift." Note, the left leg is lifted behind the musician for balance. His head is up and he is bending at his hip joint. His back remains straight and safe during the lift.

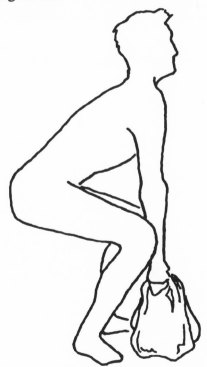

Fig.13. The weight lifter. To lift a heavy weight, keep the weight close to your body. Keep your head up and your back slightly arched. Lift with your legs.

drops his end of the weight, the other person is usually hurt.

To retrieve a ball, golfers lean on a club, lifting a leg behind them for balance and bend right over on the other leg until they can reach the ball – all without bending the low back. This is an excellent way to retrieve fairly light objects from the floor by putting one hand on something steady for balance (see photo 12, p. 67). Waiters, too, have perfected a safe lift for light objects. They bend forward from the hips, keeping their backs slightly arched and their heads up, to see if you would like a little more pasta.

Lifting anything while sitting is particularly hazardous for your low back. First, you are in a stressful position (sitting), then you must lean forward to reach whatever you intend to lift from the floor, thus losing your lordosis.

By far the most dangerous lift is when you add a body twist to a sitting lift, as when sitting in the front seat of a car and twisting around to lift an object from the floor behind your seat. If discs could scream, the noise would be deafening. Never sit, twist and lift.

Protecting Your Neck

To protect your neck while lifting an object, the same rules apply. Maintain your neck's lordosis. If you watch Olympic weight lifters' techniques, you will notice that they lift their heads up and face straight forward *before* they start to lift and *never* bend their heads forward to look down until the weights are safely back on the ground (see fig. 13, p. 67). So, if you remember to lift your head before you actually lift your child or your cello and keep it up until you have placed them somewhere else, your neck is protected. Plan ahead. If you need to carry a heavy object some distance, clear the way so that you will not need to look down sharply to avoid falling over something. Also, learn to use your eyes more and your neck less for looking down. This really takes practice and is well taught by Feldenkreis instructors.

When you have to lift anything in an awkward or difficult position, where it is impossible to keep your low back or neck in a protective lordosis, you need another approach. Before attempting the lift, bend your back and neck backward about ten times to squeeze the gel in each disc as far forward as possible (see photo 13, p. 69).

You then have a short period of time in which you can lift your suitcase off the carousel or your child out of his bathtub, before the gel is squeezed backward again by your poor lifting technique. To be safe, it is a good idea to repeat the back bends again, thus sandwiching a potentially dangerous activity between two beneficial exercises. It only takes 10 seconds to do this exercise and it may save you weeks of pain and discomfort.

To give your back a treat after a grueling day, try lying on your front as

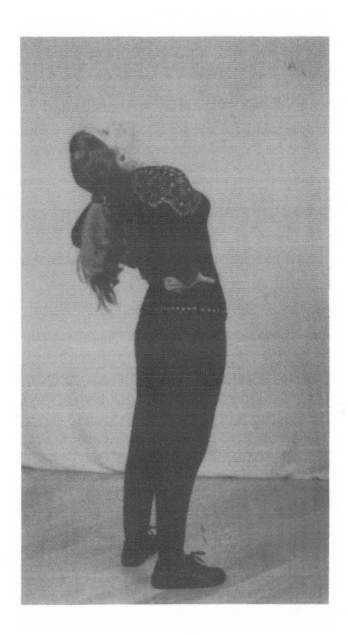

Photo 13. Bend backward before and after lifting something.

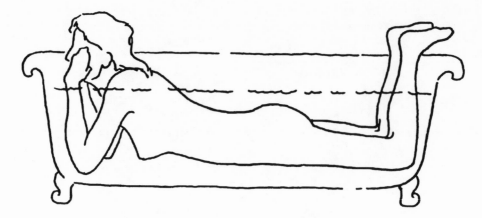

Fig. 14. Relaxing in the bathtub and giving your tired back a treat.

you soak in your bathtub, with your feet up beside the taps. If you have lost a lot of flexibility you should perhaps try this with a friend around. (The fire department does rescue people stuck in their bathtubs, but it is probably a very embarrassing experience.)

Chapter 7

The Shoulder

Anatomy

The shoulder is described as a "ball and socket" joint. The ball is on the top of the arm bone or humerus and the socket, a small, slightly curved dish, is high on the outer edge of the shoulder blade or scapula (see photo 14, p. 72).

A fibrous cuff or collar, called the labrum, is attached around the edge of the socket and deepens the socket by about 70 percent. Despite the labrum, it is still a very shallow socket and is much smaller than the head of the humerus. This allows the arm to move very freely, so that the hand can usually reach any part of the body and those who play tennis are able to serve over arm and swimmers can swim freestyle (see photo 16, p. 73).

The joint is enclosed in a capsule, which is like a fine, soft, leather bag lubricated on the inside. This capsule has a relatively large fold underneath the joint, which is stretched out when the arm is raised above the head. Woven into the capsule are ligaments and several small muscles which arise from the shoulder blade and reach across like fingers on a hand, to insert into the top of the arm bone close to the ball. These little muscles hold the ball against the socket and work hard to keep it centrally positioned there when larger muscles move the arm about. Collectively these small muscles are called the rotator cuff muscles (see photo 15, p. 72).

An arm is heavy and requires a large, strong muscle to lift it up. This muscle, the deltoid muscle, can easily be identified on anyone who develops it by weight lifting exercises, or by working with arms lifted away from the body, such as a house painter, a flautist, a conductor or a violinist (see fig. 15, p. 80). Muscles attached around the shoulder joint and inserting into the arm just below the elbow, to bend and stretch the elbow, are easily identified in anyone who performs that movement repeatedly. The biceps is on the front of the upper arm (see fig. 16, p. 80) and the triceps is on the back (see photo 17, p. 75). All of these strong muscles have one function in common. They all pull the arm bone upward in the shoulder socket, so that when you lift a heavy suitcase or instrument case, the shoulder does not dislocate downward. Their pull upward is supposed to be perfectly matched by gravity, the weight of the arm and the downward pull

71

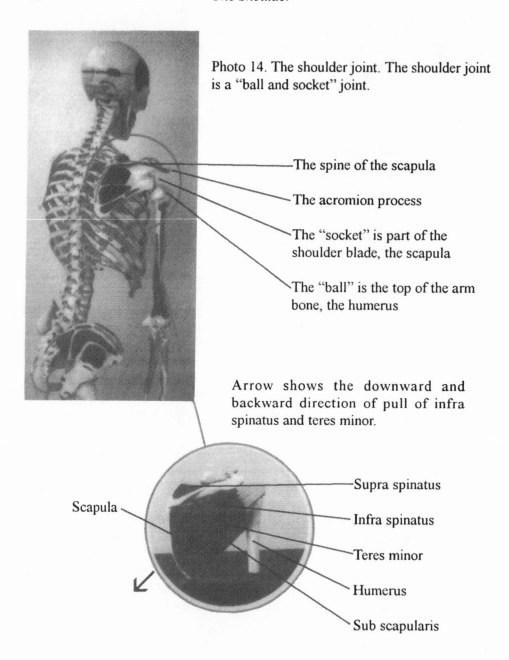

Photo 14. The shoulder joint. The shoulder joint is a "ball and socket" joint.

The spine of the scapula

The acromion process

The "socket" is part of the shoulder blade, the scapula

The "ball" is the top of the arm bone, the humerus

Arrow shows the downward and backward direction of pull of infra spinatus and teres minor.

Supra spinatus

Infra spinatus

Scapula

Teres minor

Humerus

Sub scapularis

Photo 15. The rotator cuff muscles. The rotator cuff muscles come from the shoulder blade and hold up the top of the arm bone against the socket.

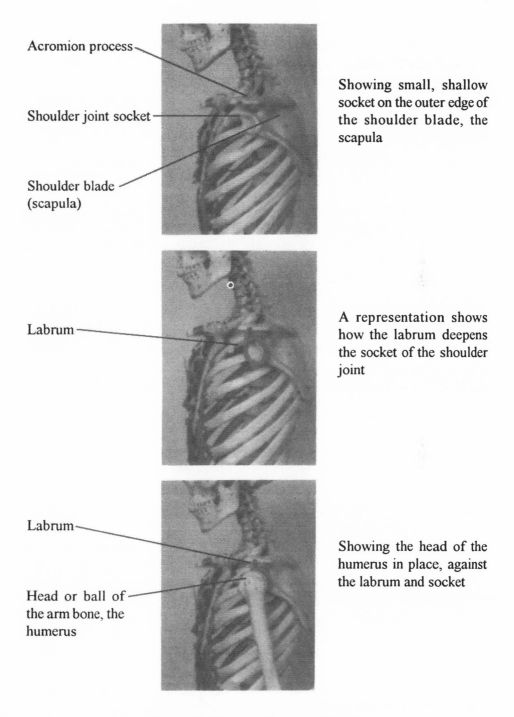

Acromion process

Shoulder joint socket

Shoulder blade
(scapula)

Showing small, shallow socket on the outer edge of the shoulder blade, the scapula

Labrum

A representation shows how the labrum deepens the socket of the shoulder joint

Labrum

Head or ball of the arm bone, the humerus

Showing the head of the humerus in place, against the labrum and socket

Photo 16. Shoulder joint and labrum.

of two of the little rotator cuff muscles, called *infra spinatus* and *teres minor* (see photo 15, p. 72) The arrow shows the direction of pull.

Muscle Imbalance

Inevitably, when string musicians in particular play a lot, their *deltoid*, *biceps* and *triceps* muscles become overdeveloped and very strong. Add to this the big muscle that pulls the arm across the front of the chest, called the pectoral muscle (see fig. 16, p. 80), and you can see that the small rotator cuff muscles are soon fighting a losing battle in their attempt to keep the top of the arm bone centered against the socket of the shoulder joint. Gradually, the ball will start to be repositioned too high and too far forward. *Infra spinatus* and *teres minor*, still trying to pull the arm bone downward and backward, become overstretched, weakened and ineffective.

This state of affairs is called *muscle imbalance* (see photo 18, p. 75) In musicians it is caused by excessive playing, not by faulty technique or tense playing. As in Christine's case, it can lead to a painful *shoulder impingement syndrome* and eventually an inability to play (see photo 20, p. 77). Muscle imbalances around the shoulders also change normal posture. The strong chest muscles become tighter and shorter and tend to pull the arms forward and turned inward, so that the hands, instead of hanging down in line with the side seams of your pants, palms facing inward, now hang in front of the thighs with the palms facing backward. This is often demonstrated by powerful, professional ball players and weight lifters who strengthen every muscle except the ones they cannot see, the rotator cuff muscles (see photo 18, p. 75).

Shoulder Impingement Syndrome

If you examine the anatomy of the shoulder even more closely, you can see that the rotator cuff muscles originating on the back of the shoulder blade are divided by a raised ridge or spine on that bone. The little muscle coming from above that spine is predictably called *supra spinatus* and it reaches across the top of the ball before holding onto the arm bone toward the front. Above the shoulder joint, the spine of the shoulder blade expands to form a ledge called the acromion process which joins with the collar bone in front and another bony protuberance from the front of the shoulder blade by means of a thick, strong, fibrous ligament (see photo 19, p. 76 and photo 20, p. 77).

The supra spinatus muscle travels through this rigid tunnel to reach the arm bone and is cushioned and protected by a bursa (a small, fluid-filled sac) from the large, bony acromion above. This mechanism works very well when the arm is lifted, until a muscle imbalance situation occurs. Once the ball of the joint

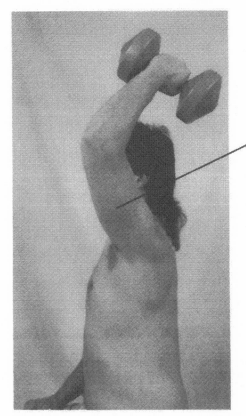

Triceps muscle

Note: this is not a recommended exercise for musicians.

Photo 17. A common free weight exercise used to strengthen triceps muscles.

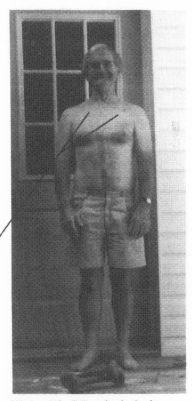

Note how this man's strong pectoral muscles have pulled his arms forward until his hands are positioned over the front of his thighs and facing backward instead of down his sides.

Photo 18. Muscle imbalances around the shoulder joint.

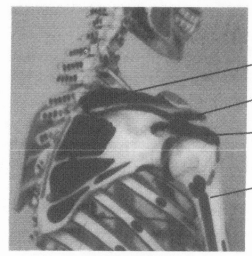

Supra spinatus muscle

Acromion process

Supra spinatus tendon holding onto
the head of the humerus

Humerus or arm bone

Side view

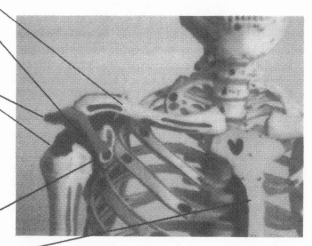

Collar bone, clavicle

Strong unyielding ligament

Acromion process

Supra spinatus tendon
coming through the narrow
rigid tunnel to reach its
insertion into the top of the
humerus

Bony protuberance from
the shoulder blade

Sternum, chest bone

Front view

Photo 19. Model of supra spinatus muscle and tendon.

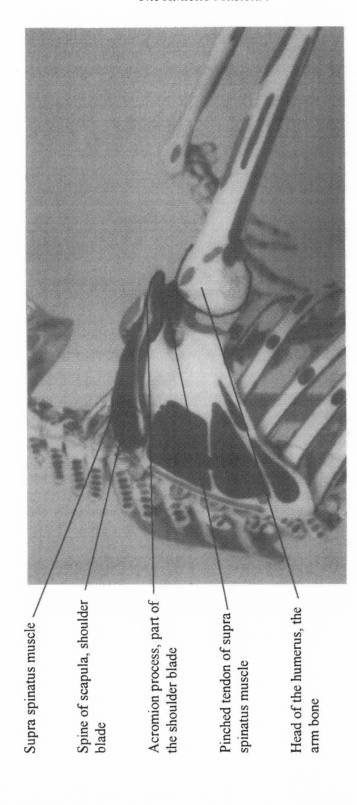

Supra spinatus muscle

Spine of scapula, shoulder blade

Acromion process, part of the shoulder blade

Pinched tendon of supra spinatus muscle

Head of the humerus, the arm bone

Photo 20. Shoulder impingement syndrome. This shows how the supra spinatus tendon is pinched or impinged between the acromion process and the head of the humerus. This happens when the ball is too high in the socket and the arm is then lifted to play.

has moved too high in the socket, every time the arm is lifted up the supra spinatus tendon is pinched against the acromion about halfway through the movement – almost exactly where a string player's bow arm spends a lot of time (see photo 21, p. 83).

Repeated pinching causes the supra spinatus tendon to become inflamed and swollen. There is certainly no room for swelling where it passes through the rigid arch and the pain increases, spreading all over the deltoid area at the top of the arm. If the musician continues to play, the pain worsens and may spread down the arm as far as the wrist. It does not spread upward into the neck, nor does the pain ever reach the hand.

By now, the musician cannot lie on that shoulder at night and will frequently continue to hurt even when not playing. Any overhead activity, like brushing hair or taking off a pullover, increases the pain immediately. Many musicians at this stage will resort to taking medication, either painkillers or anti-inflammatories, in order to continue playing. This is not a sensible thing to do, because medication only masks the pain and the injury is increased without your body being able to alert you to this by making you feel more pain. These injuries have physical, mechanical causes and therefore cannot be cured by chemical means such as pills. Recent statistics presented by Dr. Dinesh Kumbhare at Sport Med '94, a large sports medicine symposium in Toronto, alerted doctors and physiotherapists to the fact that between 3 percent and 5 percent of patients taking anti-inflammatory drugs suffer stomach reactions sufficiently severe to need hospitalization. One in 1,000 die. There seemed to be grave doubts about their effectiveness, so why take the risk?

Passive Treatments

Passive treatments such as massage, "adjustments," manipulations, acupuncture, dietary changes, reflexology, heat, ice, magnets, electricity, vitamins, copper bracelets, and so forth, may give short-term or momentary pain relief, which is certainly better than nothing. However, these treatments often result in an unhealthy long-term dependency, as they cannot provide a cure for an injury caused by muscle imbalance and overwork.

Continuing to play at this stage of the injury takes great determination and the injury is almost guaranteed to get worse if you do. Pain decreases the strength of the little rotator cuff muscles, so they become less and less able to hold the shoulder joint in the correct position. Consequently, the muscle imbalance and the impingement syndrome increase.

Now the bursa above the inflamed supra spinatus muscle is also being pinched whenever the arm is lifted up and it, too, becomes angry and inflamed.

This is called an "acute bursitis" and is so incredibly painful that even the most fanatical musician cannot bear to move the arm, and certainly cannot play. Christine described this stage well.

Because we heal, sometimes in spite of ourselves, once the shoulder is allowed to rest and is no longer irritated by valiant attempts to continue playing, the inflammation will slowly subside. *However, unless the problem of muscle imbalance is addressed and rectified, resuming playing will only result in a recurrence.*

Prevention of Muscle Imbalance around the Shoulder

Once you appreciate the anatomy of the shoulder and the muscles which activate and control arm movements, it should be obvious that certain exercises should be avoided like the plague. Strengthening deltoid, pectoral, biceps and triceps muscles by lifting weights (see figs. 15, 16, p. 80 & photos 17, 18, p. 75), or using upper body gym equipment, is going to hasten the onset of an impingement syndrome in any string musician, flautist or conductor. Even strengthening the "lats" or latissimus dorsi muscles should be avoided, as these very powerful back muscles also turn the upper arm inward and increasingly stretch and strain the rotator cuff muscles. Anyone who works with arms held away from the body has no need for any upper body strengthing exercises, because just holding the arms up creates a continuous weight lifting situation. Most musicians when tested have excellent arm, shoulder and grip strength in every muscle they continually use, exactly like every practicing athlete.

However, they generally demonstrate weakness in the two small muscles they do not use, but consistently overstretch, strain and eventually weaken. These are the infra spinatus and teres minor muscles (see photo 15, p. 72). Injury prevention protocols should therefore be aimed at first reducing the stress on these two muscles, and then strengthening them to the same level as the muscles used for playing. These little rotator cuff muscles will then be able to hold the ball of the arm bone down in the socket when the arm is lifted up to play, and impingement of supra spinatus will not occur.

To decrease postural stresses, correct your posture at all times. Stand to play whenever possible. Stand with excellent, proud posture as described previously. Lift the large bone, the sternum (see photo 19, p. 76, front view, and fig. 16, p. 80), at the front of your chest, so that your shoulders cannot droop forward. Your arms, when relaxed, should hang down by the sides of your body. Play in this erect, proud position, moving around as much as you can to avoid the fatigue of static posture. Sitting posture should be as similar to this standing position as possible. Good posture takes the strain off the rotator cuff muscles immediately, and they will soon regain some strength as a direct result of posture

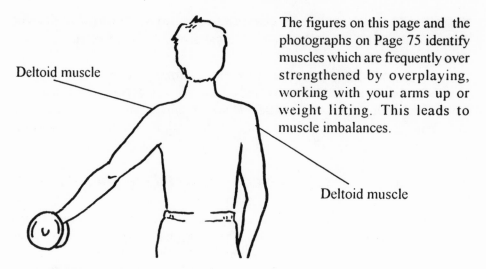

Deltoid muscle

The figures on this page and the photographs on Page 75 identify muscles which are frequently over strengthened by overplaying, working with your arms up or weight lifting. This leads to muscle imbalances.

Deltoid muscle

Fig. 15. Common free weight exercise used to strengthen deltoid muscles.

Note: these exercises are not recommended for musicians.

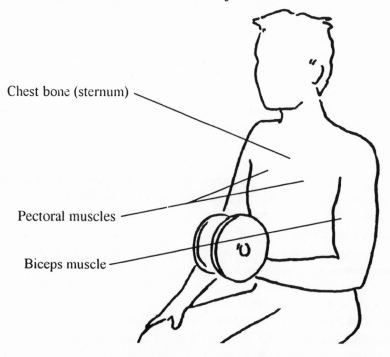

Chest bone (sternum)

Pectoral muscles

Biceps muscle

Fig. 16. Common free weight exercise to strengthen biceps muscles.

correction alone. Strengthening exercises will be described in detail in Chapter 10 addressing exercise protocols.

Thoracic Outlet or Inlet Syndrome

In my opinion this is an overused diagnosis. So far, in thirty years of practice, I have never found it in a musician. It occurs when the shoulders are dragged downward by repeatedly carrying heavy weights, or it can be caused by continuously holding the head bent right over to touch one shoulder. I have only encountered it in one man, who kept his head in this position for months to gain attention after a whiplash injury, and then again in a heavily built, middle-aged bag lady. In a thoracic outlet syndrome, there is no pain in the neck or the muscles between the neck and shoulder. Symptoms described in the arm or hand are changes in sensation, color, strength or temperature.

There is no foolproof scientific test to guarantee the existence of a thoracic outlet syndrome, and it is generally diagnosed when no other reason can be found for the strange sensations or circulatory changes reported by patients in their arms and hands. Most common tests for thoracic outlet syndrome give positive results in a large percentage of normal people, so are not much help.

Dr. James Cyriax, the father of soft tissue injuries' diagnosis, describes thoracic outlet syndrome as a "release phenomenon," meaning that the symptoms usually become more severe when the patient rests or lies down. The only useful corrective exercise is to hold the shoulders hunched up to work, play or when lifting weights. Most musicians spend a lot of time trying to stay out of that tense position, so thoracic outlet syndrome seems unlikely to be a common playing-induced complaint. It could possibly be caused by carrying a heavy instrument about all day, in which case the sensible thing to do is to rest it on your hip, put it on wheels, or get help from a stronger friend.

Contemplating removal of the first rib for relief of thoracic outlet syndrome makes this physiotherapist very nervous. If the surgeon approaches the rib from underneath, and the large nerves to the arm and hand cross over the top of that rib, the surgeon cannot see them while he is operating. There is little room for error. Any musician considering this surgery would be well advised to ask for more than one opinion, as well as a detailed description of a "worst-case" scenario. Ask for outcome statistics. How many musicians have resumed normal playing careers after this surgery? As it is not a life or death situation (although it may seem to be to musicians) there is time for contemplation and research. Talk to other musicians who have already undergone this surgery before signing consent forms. Be an informed customer.

Chapter 8

The Arm, Wrist, and Hand

Pain which occurs in the arm or hand while playing should never be ignored. If there is no history of direct injury or trauma and you are not overworking, you should not experience arm or hand pain while playing. Your body is trying to get your attention because it is being hurt. You should immediately seek help because chronic or long-standing pain is usually more difficult to relieve.

Pain in the Arm

Arm pain above the elbow can be referred from a pinched nerve in the neck or from a shoulder problem. Arm pain around or below the elbow can also be referred from the neck or shoulder, but is frequently due to faulty wrist positioning or overuse of wrist movements while playing.

Arm pain down the back of the forearm often starts just above the outside bony point of the elbow. It is very similar to tennis elbow in athletes and has a similar cause. The culprit is in fact the wrist joint and again we must examine the anatomy. If you look at the position your wrist adopts when you make a fist or grip an object very firmly, you will see the so-called "neutral position" where the wrist performs best. Now let your hand bend forward at the wrist, so that the palm of your hand moves toward the front of your forearm. This is called wrist flexion (see photo 22, p. 83). Here, the muscles which originate at the elbow and stretch down the back of the forearm to move your fingers are on full stretch. Doing this movement as a pre- and postplaying stretch is fine, but prolonged working or playing in this position is asking for trouble in the back of the forearm, and elbow and hand. Try to make a fist with your wrist in flexion and you will see and feel the lack of power and strength in your hand.

Pain in the Elbow

The easiest way to strain an elbow joint is to carry something too heavy, so that the joint is pulled very straight. Very heavy suitcases will do this to you, as

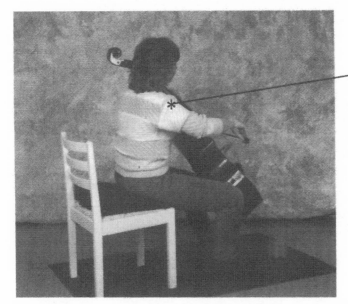

Impingement pain is usually felt here when the bow arm is in this horizontal position.

Photo 21. Shoulder impingement position.

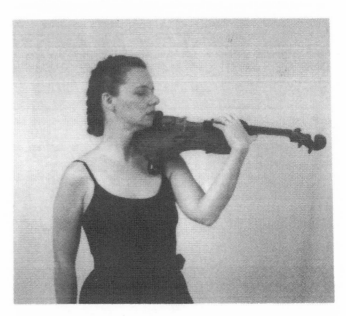

Photo 22. Violinist demonstrates left wrist's flexion position.

will moving furniture or carrying too many bags full of groceries. Elbows have a "carrying angle," which means they like to stay slightly bent when carrying things comfortably. It is a good idea to respect that carrying angle and protect this very complex joint from harm. Should any musician, or indeed anyone else, be so unfortunate as to sustain a serious injury or fracture in the elbow region, do not treat it lightly, as elbows can react alarmingly to poor orthopedic management, and your hand needs a fully mobile elbow to be able to play most instruments.

Pain in the Wrist

Musicians, like tennis players and golfers, need to pay attention to their wrist positions while playing and avoid overusing wrist movements. We see these problems most frequently in guitarists and harpists, who strum or pluck the strings using repeated wrist movements, as well as in pianists, who sit too low – but there are many more. *Wrist flexion is invariably the position or overused movement which will cause trouble for all musicians, athletes and workers* (see photos 23, 24, 25, pp. 85-87).

Pain in the Hand

Hand pain is usually due to abuse or overuse. Hands are designed to work hard and have many small, strong muscles in the palm and around the thumb which thrive on activity. As with all muscles, they need to be warm to play and need gentle warm-up and cool-down exercises and stretches before and after a hard workout. They do best with varied activities, not the same difficult movement repeated over and over again. They appreciate *frequent rests* for recuperation and frequent relief from being in weird positions. As with all other joints in the body, finger joints like movement. They object to being stressed or strained at the extreme of any movement, and will react with pain if you hold your instrument by pushing any finger or thumb joint as far as it will go and keeping it there – be that bent, straightened or twisted (see photo 29, p. 102). You can test this reaction easily by simply stretching one of your fingers backward, away from the palm and applying overpressure with your other hand. The stretched finger joints will soon transmit pain signals, asking you to stop.

If you keep your fingers and thumb slightly curved, as when holding a coffee mug, they will tolerate holding objects more easily, so keep that analogy in mind if you are making modifications to your instrument (see photo 26, p. 92).

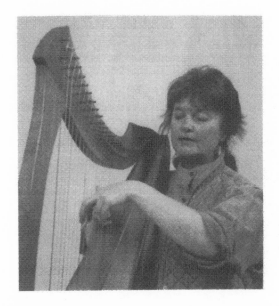

Overuse of this wrist flexion movement frequently causes
arm and hand pain.

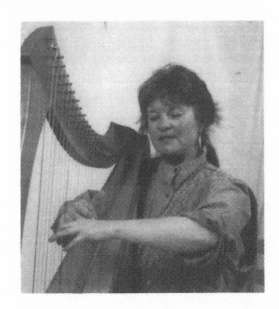

A good neutral wrist position.

Photo 23. Harpist demonstrates wrist positions.

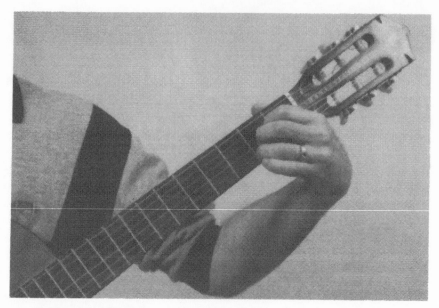

Avoid overusing this wrist flexion position.

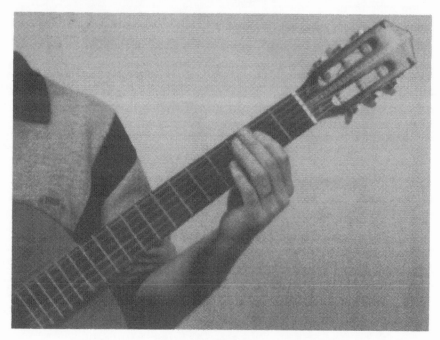

Demonstrating a good, neutral position.

Photo 24. Guitarist demonstrates wrist positions.

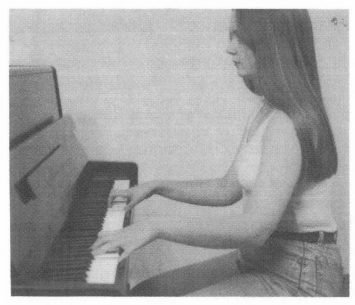

Sitting on a low bench, this pianist plays in wrist flexion.
This frequently leads to arm or hand pain.

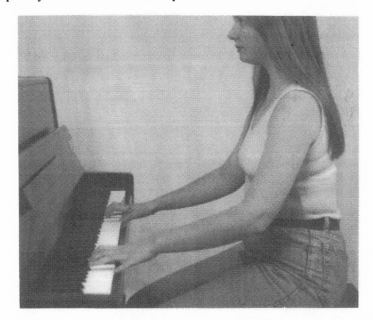

On a higher seat, she is able to play with her wrist in a
safe, neutral position.

Photo 25. Pianist demonstrates wrist positions.

Overwork

If you seriously overwork your hands, or use them as jackhammers in a rigid posture for repeated traumatic attacks upon the piano, you can cause pain that spreads from the palms up the front of the forearms to the front of the elbows. It really does not make sense to abuse your hands in such a manner. Habitual overplaying can cause serious damage to tendons and nerves in the hands and wrists, frequently spreading into the forearms.

The pain induced by overplaying indicates that either a nerve in your forearm, wrist or hand is being compressed, or that small muscles in the palm or finger tendons have been strained. The musician receives several warning signs of impending overuse injuries and should take them seriously, as they can affect future playing abilities if allowed to become chronic conditions. As well as pain being experienced while playing or immediately after playing, the hands and/or forearms feel swollen, tight and heavier than usual. There are frequently complaints of decreased dexterity, i.e., dropping an occasional note or two.

What is happening? Repeated, overvigorous finger movements can strain the small muscles inside the palm of the hand. These will recover with rest and a few treatment sessions.

Finger Tendons

Finger tendons, however, are a different matter. Long tendons go from muscles in the front of the forearms to bend your finger joints. They glide through well-lubricated tendon sheaths which provide nourishment and protect the tendons where they pass over the wrist and finger bones. There is sufficient lubrication in these sheaths for normal hand use and it is replenished during breaks in activity. If you play for too many hours or for too long without breaks, these sheaths run out of lubrication and the tendons will rub inside the sheaths, causing irritation, inflammation, swelling and pain. This is similar to making your car engine run without oil. The pistons would soon stop gliding up and down the cylinders and the surfaces would soon be damaged. This situation calls for immediate rest from playing for at least a day or two. Thinking like an athlete, use ice packs for the pain and swelling and gently move the finger occasionally to promote healing and to prevent any scarring between the tendons and their protective sheaths. Do not do strengthening exercises for overworked hands or arms or you will get worse instead of better. Instead, start walking more or swimming, cycling etc., using your legs to improve your overall health and conditioning, to help your body recover. Practice only in your head. Brains store your ability to play and they do not get tendonitis or tenosynovitis.

Continuing to overwork and overpractice, ignoring your hands' needs and warning signs, can lead to career-threatening, chronic tendonitis. This is where the tendons in your hands and wrists are trying to glide through tendon sheaths that are now thickened and chronically inflamed or scarred. The smooth, lubricated, gliding movements and good tendon nutrition provided by the lubricating fluid in the tendon sheaths are all compromised. Treatment is long term and not always successful.

Nerve Symptoms in the Hand

Nerve symptoms in the hand feel different from the pain of overused muscles. The sensations can be pain, pins and needles, numbness or tingling and finger strength and coordination can be affected.

Again, the symptoms can be referred from the neck, elbow or wrist, so it is important to obtain a differential diagnosis through a careful examination of each area by your orthopedic physiotherapist. Simple, precise testing of joint movements and positions, muscle strength, reflexes and skin sensation is usually sufficient to pinpoint the cause of the problem. Electromyographic (EMG) studies should be saved for unusual cases, or for problems which do not respond quickly or as expected to treatment protocols.

Occupational Injuries

Drawing from copious amounts of data accumulated by health and safety associations investigating soft tissue injuries in industry, musicians can identify similar risk factors. Workers who use their hand and arm muscles very forcefully, with many repeated, fast-paced movements, suffer from rapid muscle fatigue. They frequently need rest periods that must exceed the actual time worked if they are to avoid accumulative muscle or tendon trauma. The likelihood of injury is increased if their work necessitates adopting awkward neck postures, such as bending or twisting. Working with one or both arms held away from the body, without any support for the weight of the arms is similarly identified as hazardous posture.

Repeatedly lifting the arms out to the side, repeatedly twisting the forearms and frequently working with the wrists flexed forward (palm bending toward the forearm) or deviated outward (hands bending toward the fifth finger) are all activities and positions that have been identified as responsible for accumulative wear and tear injuries that stop the workers from being able to do their jobs. Working in cold conditions, where workers actually feel cold while they work, increases their susceptibility to injury.

Obviously, some work does include some of these hazardous components, so industrial health and safety experts have recommended a *two-hour limit* for each of these continuous activities, followed by either adequate rest or a complete change of activity, i.e., job rotations. Workers whose jobs include five of the above activities or positions and who do not take the required rest breaks are identified as being at *high risk* of occupational injury.

Reading this, I am sure many musicians are comparing themselves with the workers on the high-risk list. It would be reasonable to use this industrial information and advice to prevent playing injuries. If for some reason you simply cannot improve your playing ergonomics or posture, at least keep warm! Two hours of concentrated practicing should be your self-imposed limit for safety. From what we have learned from athletes, this would be a good time to practice the art of "mental practice." Find somewhere quiet to lie down, close your eyes, relax your tired muscles and then, only in your mind, return to your instrument and spend time playing the music you practiced all over again. (See p. 136 re: mental practice and suggestions on p. 144.)

Syndromes

Arm and hand injuries are frequently assigned group names, e.g., carpal tunnel syndrome (CTS), repetitive strain injury (RSI), thoracic outlet syndrome (TOS), or cumulative trauma disorder (CTD). Before agreeing to have any "syndrome," insist upon a thorough clinical examination and at least one second opinion if there is any doubt. Each "syndrome" requires a very different treatment approach, and it is most annoying if your carpel tunnel syndrome does not respond to weeks of wrist therapy or desperation-driven surgery because it was in fact a neck problem.

Repetitive strain injury is also too vague a term to be acceptable. I recently attended an international pain symposium in Vancouver, BC, where medical experts from Europe, Great Britain, Australia and North America presented RSI as a "regional pain syndrome" (RPS) affecting injured people who suffered primarily from psychosocial distress. As musicians generally experience psychosocial distress as a result of suffering from a playing injury and being unable to play, the chicken and egg syndrome (C&ES) here is important. If these pain experts truly reflected present international thinking about RSI, musicians would do well to request a more specific anatomical diagnosis, naming the strained muscle, joint or tendon involved and disassociate themselves from RSI as a catch-all diagnosis. As soon as there is any hint that a condition or syndrome could be psychosocially induced or prolonged, this is a tempting straw to be grasped by any health professional who cannot help you. "When all else fails, blame the patient."

Another problem with vague, general terms like RSI and TOS is that they have been known to receive equally vague, nonspecific treatment, as likely to irritate the injured tissue as to relieve it. A general exercise program appropriate for a regional pain syndrome type of RSI is certainly not appropriate treatment for a musician's specific muscle, tendon or nerve injury. The best that can happen is that the injury will heal without help. The worst scenario is that the general exercise and weight lifting routines can regularly irritate the injured tissues sufficiently to prevent natural healing from occurring. If you have been faithfully exercising for several months and still hurt when you play, you may wish to question the value of your exercises. Musicians need specific injury treatment and should not be subjected to the type of general fitness programs designed to combat chronic pain syndromes (where injuries and pathology have been ruled out as a reason for the continuing pain).

Injured athletes certainly work hard on individually designed exercise programs which enable them to maintain their desired level of fitness while protecting their injuries. These injuries meanwhile receive specific physiotherapy care, ensuring that the healing occurs while normal movement and flexibility is restored. Applying the correct amount of stress at the right stage of healing is crucial if any injury is to heal with strong, flexible, resilient tissue. Mindless, general exercise routines cannot accomplish this. Nor can nonmedical practitioners prescribe safe, effective exercise protocols for injured people. (See Chapter 14 for information on various health care providers.)

Wrist and Hand Splints

The use of wrist and hand splints is controversial, but they can be useful devices when used appropriately. For example, a brace can be used to support and protect a hand injury such as saxophone or oboe player's thumb (see photo 27, p. 92) until the musician has investigated alternative ways to take the weight of the instrument. Thumbs were not designed to carry weight this way.

A temporary wrist brace can be used to stop or retrain overused or faulty wrist movements. A cellist told me she remembered her teacher strapping a ruler to the inside of her forearm and wrist to prevent her overusing wrist movements as a child. This sounds a bit draconian (Christine was horrified!) but she says it soon had the desired effect. Finding a wrist brace which will hold the wrist joint in neutral, without inhibiting normal hand function or altering how you use the rest of your arm and hand, has presented quite a challenge. There is no perfect brace that will suit everyone. General guidelines are that the brace must be snug but comfortable and must have sufficient built-in strength to prohibit the faulty movement. There are many designs and manufacturers, so consult your occupational or physical therapist.

If you simply cannot play in a wrist brace, but your wrist is causing trouble, consider wearing a brace to control wrist movements when you are not playing.

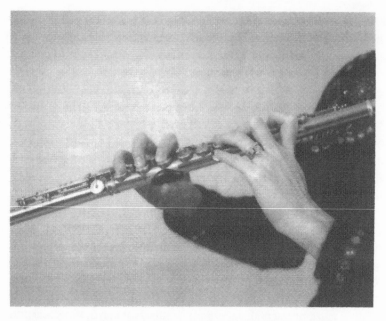

Photo 26. Improving the position of the right thumb by adding
width to the flute with a Bo-Pep™ thumb guide™.

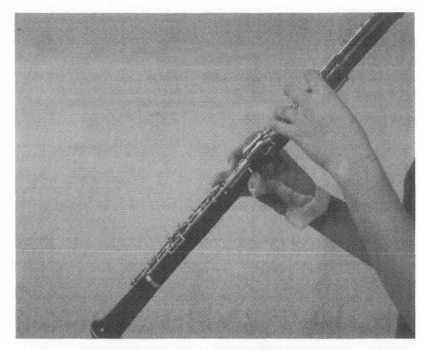

Photo 27. Using custom-made thumb splint to support weight
of the oboe.

For example, a young cello player complained that a previous wrist injury was again giving her trouble. She was practicing several hours each evening after working all day as a landscape gardener, planting small plants by hand. A wrist support while she planted prevented repetitive wrist motions and she could then tolerate playing without the brace in the evenings. Similarly, people who sleep with their hands and wrists tucked into bent "praying mantis" positions may have to use wrist braces at night to avoid this, if they waken with any changes of sensation in their hands.

Occupational and physical therapists working in hospital hand clinics are very helpful to consult about protective bracing for finger or thumb injuries. They will custom-make braces to protect any hurt joint or ligament in the hand or wrist and will advise how and when to use them. Generally speaking, fingers are so prone to healing stiff that one aims for short-term rigid splinting of any kind for hand sprains and strains. Sprained thumb muscles and tendons seem to respond best to short-term immobilization. Wearing braces on your hands or wrists when you are suffering from overuse or overplaying injuries needs careful management by a physiotherapist or occupational therapist.

There is no splint or brace to prevent changes in sensation in the fourth and fifth fingers (see p. 30) and the side of the hand when it is due to pressure on the nerve at the elbow's "funny bone." In daytime, simply stop resting your elbow on hard surfaces. At night, you may have to fasten your arms down by your sides (as it is usually caused by lying face down with arms above your head), so that the nerve and inside bone at the elbow are pressed onto the bed by the weight of your relaxed arm. If that does not fix it, you need help to find the real cause, which could be anywhere from the neck to the hand.

PART III

The Musician as Athlete

Chapter 9

Playing Ergonomics

Ergonomics and the Musician

The *Oxford Dictionary* defines ergonomics as "the relationship between people and their working environment, as it effects efficiency, safety and ease of action...." For musicians, playing ergonomics deals with how musicians and their instruments and equipment relate to each other in these terms.

Musicians have always been concerned with the efficiency of their instruments. We spend countless hours and lots of money making sure that they sound as good as they possibly can. We go to great lengths to ensure that our instruments, as entities separate from ourselves, function with "ease of action." Historically, most of our focus has been on the affect or impact we have on our instruments and not on how our instruments affect us. The ergonomic relationship between player and instrument has been one-sided: whenever one must adapt to the other, it is usually the musician who does the adapting. Paganini is a great example of this. When they dug up his skeleton, it was discovered that the left shoulder, which had supported the violin for so many years, was several inches higher than the right. If you'd like to prove this point to yourself and don't have any ex-violinist friends waiting to be exhumed, just walk behind a group of string players at your next rehearsal break and see how many of them have grown around their instruments in the same way.

If musicians worked in a factory environment with heavy equipment and complex machinery, we would be very concerned with the ergonomics of our equipment as it related to our health and safety. If we worked at computer terminals in an office and were entitled to sick pay and disability benefits, our employers would be very concerned with the ergonomics of our computer set-up as related to employee health. Our focus with musical instruments is different, yet statistically we know that playing an instrument can lead to significant health problems. As most efficiency experts or ergonomists won't understand the fine points of playing an instrument, we need to be our own "ergonomists." We need to arrive at ergonomic solutions that in no way compromise either our instruments, our playing, or our health.

Despite the fact that most instruments we play today were designed centuries ago, they are not obsolete anachronisms that need to be reinvented. Advances in technology and changes in the demands of modern technique and style have resulted in a certain amount of evolution of instruments, but the basic principles of their designs are unchanged. Three hundred years ago, violin makers were producing instruments that remain unsurpassed today. Our difficulty in using these instruments to meet the demands of the twentieth century lies in the fact that they were designed to meet only acoustical and musical ideals. Knowledge of anatomy was not where it is today, and while all instruments were designed to be played, ergonomic efficiency was not the main objective.

Ergonomics and Posture

There are steps that you can take to adapt and modify instruments to be more "user friendly" without interfering with their performance or yours. Many musicians would not consider changing anything fundamental in the design of their instruments, regardless of the benefit to their health. For example, angled head joints have been designed for flutes that enable the players to maintain correct neck posture while keeping their arms lower. They make perfect sense in terms of ease of use and the anatomy, but they are not widely accepted because most flautists feel that they compromise their playing. Brass and woodwind players have modified their instruments over time by adding or moving keys, and these changes have been universally accepted because the only effect they have on playing is to make it easier. String instruments have evolved to some degree to meet the demands of modern technique (longer necks and fingerboards on violins, for example), but again, these changes did not compromise the way the instruments sound. Players are so reluctant to make any change to a string instrument that even something as universally accepted as the chin rest created a real controversy back in the mid-seventeenth century when it was introduced by Louis Sphor. Despite the sophistication of the twentieth century and all research to the contrary, there are still players today who refuse to use a shoulder rest because they believe it affects the tone of the instrument.

From the musician's point of view, any ergonomic adaptation to an instrument must not compromise the integrity of the instrument in any way, and any change to playing, even a change that makes it easier to play, must not involve a major revamping of technique. From the physiotherapists' point of view, for any ergonomic adaptation to be successful or worthwhile, it has to be based on the objectives of obtaining a posture that is as close to anatomically correct as possible, allowing joints to function in as neutral a position as possible. Any change in equipment and posture may take a bit of getting used to, but changes should ultimately result in greater ease and comfort with the instrument.

Most instruments come in "one-size-fits-all." Sometimes this explains why some players never experience problems, while others don't stand a chance with their instrument. The size of the player is not the big issue (there have been world-renowned pianists with short fingers, bulky piccolo players, petite cellists, etc.), but the shape of the player is important.

The length of your neck and shape of your shoulders can affect your neck posture when you play. For example, violinists with short necks, square shoulders and lots of natural padding can tuck their instrument under one of their many chins without having to raise a shoulder or lower their neck. Players built this way have no use for shoulder rests – they are able to maintain a straight, upright head position without one, and if they teach they may outlaw shoulder rests for all their students. Their pupils who look like them will be fine, but others with giraffe necks, small chins, narrow sloping shoulders and bony collarbones will have to play with raised shoulders and bent necks (see photo 28, p. 100). Holding a telephone between the side of your head and your raised shoulder to leave your hands free, has a similar effect upon a long neck.

The way an instrument is set up can affect posture. For instance, almost all violists use a chin rest, but how it is designed and where it is placed can affect neck posture. If the chin rest is shaped like a deep cup with a high ridge, the player has to jut her head forward and place it sideways in the chin rest so that the jaw bone doesn't sit uncomfortably on the high ridge (see photo 28, p. 100). If this same chin rest is placed on the side rather than centered over the tailpiece (depending on the width of the lower bouts and the size of the player), the player may also have to rotate his neck to get to the chin rest. This also results in the weight of the instrument lying in front of the player, rather than up on the shoulder. Chapter 5 explains why these neck positions (flexion, protraction and rotation) are undesirable.

Evaluating your Ergonomics, or How to Play the Viola without Looking Like a Pretzel

Healthy players can examine the ergonomics of their setup with the instrument. If you are injured, do not attempt this on your own. What is ideal posture for someone without injuries may be out of the question for a hurt player, and efforts to change equipment to achieve a postural ideal may end up making you worse. If you are hurt, you must work with your physiotherapist to achieve ergonomic solutions which may change as your recovery progresses. Ideally, you should work in consultation with a musician who understands what the physiotherapist is after and knows how to achieve this on the instrument.

Begin your ergonomic examination of your playing by finding out who's doing the adapting, you or the instrument. You'll need help from a teacher,

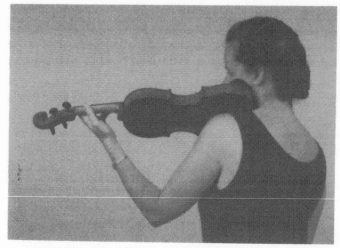

Violinist, left, adapting her head and neck to a chinrest that is shaped like a deep cup. This position leads to neck pain.

This musician, right, demonstrates how her body adapts to her instrument. Her long neck bends sideways and her left shoulder is held up high and pushed forward. This position will eventually cause neck problems.

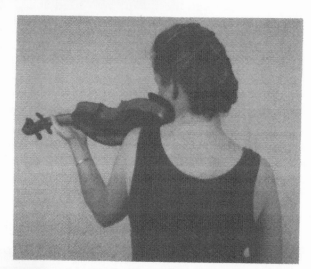

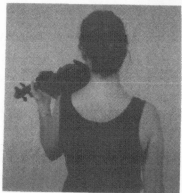

Neck and shoulder posture, left, corrected using an extra high rest.

Photo 28. Using ergonomic principles to correct a violinist's playing posture.

physiotherapist, fellow player, three-way mirror or video camera because you need to see what's going on from a number of angles.

Stand in the "athletic posture" without the instrument and look at your back view. Make sure your shoulders are "square" so your spine isn't twisted. Notice the level of your shoulders. Check the side view. Assuming you are healthy and have full neck retraction, your ears should be lined up over your shoulders. Now look at the front view. Unless you were a boxer in a previous life, your nose should be pointing straight ahead and not off to one side.

Pick up your instrument and play a bit of your favorite piece and then, still holding the instrument, take a look at yourself. What you see may surprise you, so play and check again. Starting out in the athletic posture, position the instrument again and you might witness the "magnetic viola" phenomenon. We can become so accustomed to adapting our bodies to the instrument, rather than vice versa, that as you bring the instrument up to the shoulder you may find your head going down to the viola, your neck twisting to the left, your left shoulder pushing forward and up and your upper body folding itself over and around the instrument. Check hand and wrist positions to see if you are asking any joint to stay at the end of its range of motion. If you notice anything that deviates from athletic posture and neutral joint positions, perhaps your present equipment isn't allowing you to maintain an athletic posture when you play.

Now that you know what goals you are trying to achieve, experiment with ergonomic adaptations to your instrument. For instance, flautists will likely notice that the left index finger and right thumb are held at the end of their range of motion. Rather than assuming the shape your hand would make holding a small cup (see p. 84) your right hand may have the thumb pushed in tightly to the hand. Some players have found it helpful to use a "Bo-Pep™" attachment for one or both hands (see photo 26, p. 92 and photo 29, p. 102).

Consultations with people who have experience in this area may help, but players are the only ones who can decide what will work for them. It can take a lot of trial and error, but the difference it can make in your comfort and ease with the instrument is well worth the effort.

When you think you've come up with a solution you can live with, try out your new setup while practicing at home and then perhaps at a rehearsal or concert. If you are injured and have been trying to find solutions to the cause of your problem, you'll quickly get used to any ergonomic adaptation that enables you to play without pain (rather like getting used to a pair of comfortable shoes after suffering blisters). Even if you decide that you can't adjust to postural "perfection" when you play, whatever you do to reduce harmful positions and improve poor postures will be of enormous help in keeping you injury free. If you feel more comfortable when you play, chances are you'll sound better also. Remember – what's good for your body will be good for your playing.

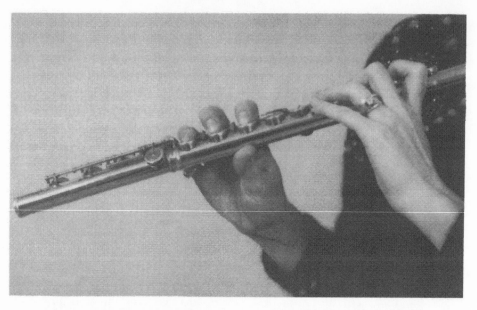

Playing with the left index finger pushed to the limit of its movement. This joint will eventually hurt.

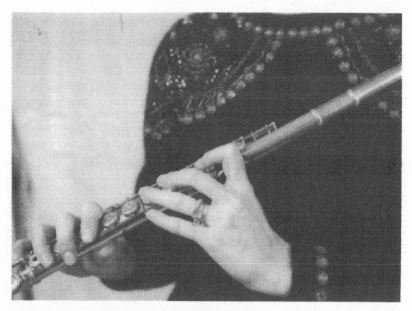

Corrected left index finger using a Bo-Pep™.

Photo 29. Flautist demonstrates how to relieve a stressful finger position.

Ergonomics and Other Equipment

Musicians need to consider how all their equipment affects them. The demands of each person's instrument and job will be different. For instance, players in a rock band who can't yet afford to hire someone else to move and set up their heavy equipment may find that they are more at risk from injury getting ready to play than they are from the actual performance. Almost all musicians will have to sit when they perform, use music stands, and carry their instruments in a case, so let's take an ergonomic look at these common areas.

Chairs

In an ideal world, every musician would have an ergonomically designed chair to work in. Until that time comes, there are a few things that you can do to adapt inadequate seating.

Barbara has talked about chairs as they relate to posture in Chapter 6. Check the height of your chair seat and if you find that your chair is too low, you can:

- put wooden blocks under the legs
- add a cushion on top of the seat, or
- stack two chairs together

The advantages of an angled seat are explained in Chapter 6. Some instrumentalists (harpists and organists, for instance, who need to keep the weight off their feet to access the pedals) may not be able to play if they are on an angle. Silk weavers in Bangkok, however, have designed an angled seat that allows them to use both feet to operate the looms (see photo 31, p. 106). Most other players would find that an angled seat helps them sit more effortlessly without negatively affecting their playing. You can carry a wedge-shaped cushion with you and use it on any chair. Another way to angle the seat is to put blocks under the back legs of your chair.

If there is nothing you can do to correct or improve your chair, at least prevent it from hurting you. Sit in such a way that you are able to stand up without shifting your weight. Perch on the edge of the chair, with one or both of your knees lower than your hips. Violinists and violists should drop the right knee so that their hand does not hit their leg when bowing on the upper strings. In this way you can avoid twisting your spine and maintain a natural lordosis in your low back. Your chest bone, the sternum, should be lifted and your head should be erect and retracted to a balanced, midline position. The edge of the seat may press into the back of your thigh a little, but your back and neck will be safe (see photo 30, p. 104).

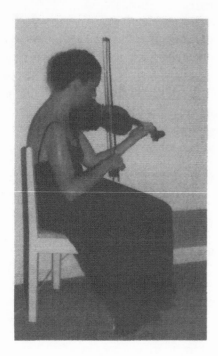

A poor playing posture, leading to back and neck ache.

Correct playing posture, right, on a poorly designed chair. the player is perched on the front of the chair. Her right knee is dropped and her right foot is under the chair. She could stand up from this position without having to move her feet.

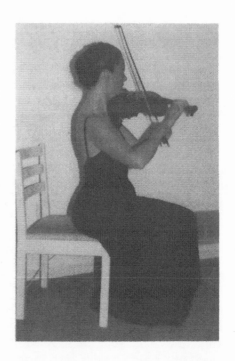

Photo 30. Violinist demonstrates how to cope with a poorly designed chair.

Music Stands

A stand should be positioned like the monitor on your home computer. Your eyes should be level with the center of the page that you're reading. This is a very simple concept, but many musicians develop neck problems because their stands are too low and they must sit with a flexed-neck position. Your setup at home should be ideal. As you will be practicing standing up whenever possible, your only problem will be finding a stand that is high enough for you if you're taller than 5'6". You may have to have something custom-made, or resort to pinning your music up with clothespins (which can make page turns difficult!). If you are traveling and don't have a stand handy, rather than propping up your music on your case and bending over to see it, try tacking it up with putty (sold in office supply stores), or sticking it in the frame of the dresser mirror.

Orchestral players need to keep their stands lower than eye level so that they can see the conductor. Brass players may face this problem if they want the bell of the instrument over the stand (see photo 32, p. 106). In this case, get the stand as high as you can, and try to look down your nose at the music, rather than bending your neck. Compensate for any neck flexion by doing the neck extension exercise whenever you can (see photo 43, p. 150).

Cases

It is surprising how many players of large, heavy instruments attribute their back problems to their playing without considering what they are doing to their bodies by constantly lifting and carrying their instruments. If you're not wealthy enough to hire someone to cart your things for you, think about adding wheels to your case. A double bass, for example, can be wheeled much easier than carried.

Most tuba players wouldn't think of trying to go shopping between rehearsals carrying their instruments. Players of smaller, lighter instruments are more likely to ignore the weight that they have become so accustomed to. Sometimes, it is only when we buy a new case that happens to be a bit lighter than our old one that we realize what a strain carrying the instrument has been. Regardless of what it does to our bodies, we are most likely to consider instrument safety above our own when we choose a case. Shop around and you may find that there are lot of options that can offer the same protection without compromising strength. If you have a heavy case or instrument, you can also try adding straps and carrying it like a back pack, or using a wheeled "airport" cart. (Luggage stores are a good source.)

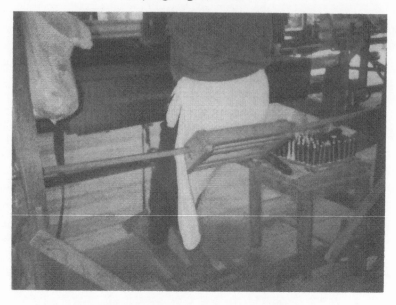

Photo 31. Bangkok silk weaver's chair.

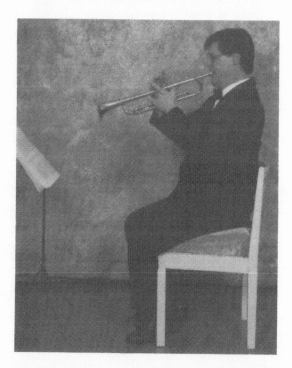

Photo 32. Trumpet player uses a wedge cushion to improve a poor chair. Note his good head posture. His music stand is as high as circumstances allow.

Ergonomics for Pianists

Pianists are at a disadvantage when it comes to making their instruments ergonomically effective, as so often they must perform on an instrument that is not their own. There are steps you can take to make sure that your own instrument is as ergonomically efficient as possible, and there are some things that can be done when you must adapt other instruments.

Piano benches need to be viewed in the same light as chairs (see Chapter 6). Some padded benches and round stools adjust for height, but most standard benches do not. If you need a bench that is higher than the standard, you may have to jack up the legs with wooden blocks. It's probably not a great idea to start sawing off pieces of the bench if it's not your own, so people who need something lower than standard are in a bit of a fix. When deciding on the optimal height of your piano bench, you need to consider how the angle of your wrist will be affected. For instance, a child or a very short adult may find that the standard height of piano bench puts their wrists into a flexed position at the keyboard (see photo 25, p. 87). The benefits of an angled seat have been discussed in Chapter 6. As piano benches are not mass produced with this feature, you may wish to experiment with a wedge cushion that you can use with any bench. Wedge cushions make it easier to maintain correct back posture and have two added advantages for the pianist: 1) they make it easier to use upper body weight when you play, and 2) they soften the sharp angle at the front edge of the standard smooth piano bench. This edge can dig into your legs, reducing circulation and putting pressure on the sciatic nerve. (If you are proficient at woodworking, you can bevel and round this edge off yourself.)

Neck posture at the piano or keyboard can be affected by the height of the music rack. If the rack is too low (as with synthesizers and most grand pianos), you may be bending your head down in an attempt to adapt your neck to the instrument, rather than vice versa. It is possible to buy attachments that will lower the music, but you may have to improvise to get your music higher. (Clothespins don't look great, but they work – until you hit a page turn.)

The majority of your practice time will likely be spent on your own instrument. Work with your piano technician to ensure that your own piano functions the way it should. Consider the following factors as they relate to the ergonomics of playing:

a. Action and weight (hammer blow and key weights)
b. Depth of touch
c. Carding
d. Voicing

Action

The actions of upright and grand pianos are mechanically different. You can't adapt an upright to work against gravity or with the same leverage system as a grand, but you can have the keys weighted to match the weight of a grand. Even among grand pianos, the weight of the keys differs, depending on the size of the piano. (The block of wood and felt from which the hammers are fashioned varies in weight from 17 to 19 pounds.) An Olympic athlete would train under conditions as close as possible to competition conditions. You need to practice on a 9-foot grand piano if you are going to be performing on one on a regular basis. If this isn't possible, work with your technician to come up with a similarly weighted action on your own piano. If your piano is used primarily to teach young children, it doesn't make sense to have the action weighted as heavily as a grand. Where you have access to more than one piano, you may wish to do some of your practicing on an instrument with a lighter action. You can have your technician check the lost action in the keys. If this "dead space" at the top of the keys is too great, you will lose hammer blow. The hammers will be striking the strings from a shorter distance and you will have to play with more force to obtain the volume you require.

Depth of Touch

Certain makes of pianos are known for a greater depth of touch than others. This encourages a feeling of sinking into the keys, rather than "bottoming out." A shallow depth of touch can lead to a more percussive technique and feel a bit like jogging on cement without good running shoes. Synthesizer players deal with this kind of action, but don't need to worry about producing the changes in volume or subtleties of tone that pianists concern themselves with. Depth of touch can usually be restored or adjusted.

Carding

If you've been playing four or five hours a day for the past two years or so and haven't had your technician card the hammers of your piano, you'll find that the strings have worn deep grooves in them. As the hammer strikes the strings, the sound is actually dampened by these deep grooves surrounding the string. The pianist has to work more to produce the same volume. Carding involves filing down the hammers to get rid of the grooves. Most technicians would agree that hammers can be carded twice before you have to consider having them replaced.

Voicing

When technicians "voice" a piano, they alter the hardness of the hammers, either chemically or manually. If the felts are too hard, the sound will be harsh and percussive; when the felts are too soft, the sound will be "woolly" and dead. Voicing is a matter of personal preference, but it is important for pianists to understand what their options are. You will be expending a lot of unnecessary effort trying to produce a sharp, brilliant tone on a piano with soft felts.

Chapter 10

Exercise Protocols for the Musical Athlete

Exercise protocols should address the whole body for general well-being and then those parts of your body you use to play. Musicians need to understand athletic definitions of warm-ups, cool-downs, stretches, strengthening exercises, general conditioning and cross-training. Aim to establish regular physical exercise routines which will help your body to stay fit, flexible and strong and counteract fatigue and the common playing-induced injuries described in previous chapters.

Some exercise protocols are presented for offstage or away from your instrument. Others are designed to help you through long practice sessions or actual performances. All of these protocols need your active participation. There are no passive treatments or magic machines that can gain the required results for you. Massage, for example, may help you to relax if you are feeling very tense and nervous, but the only person who gains strength, muscle bulk and increased aerobic capacity is the masseur!

Warm-ups

A "warm-up" means using muscles gently and smoothly for a few minutes to increase the blood flow through them without stressing them. Your muscles should always be warmed up in preparation for stretching and working as cold muscles simply will not stretch. Physically, you should feel comfortably warm to work or exercise, so wear adequate clothing if you are in a cold place.

To warm up your whole body take a short, brisk walk or jog, or trot up and down the stairs a few times. Turn on your radio and dance to some medium-paced music for a few minutes. Warm-ups should make you feel energized, not exhausted, and should not leave you short of breath.

To warm up your arms and shoulders before playing, swing your arms as if marching, then do about ten repeated self-hugs and releases.

To warm up your wrists and hands, you can either mime a thorough washing with soap and water, or massage real or imaginary hand lotion into your hands and fingers.

Stretching

Stretching is done for two main reasons. One is to maintain flexibility or full movements in your joints, and the other is to maintain your muscles' full extensibility or ability to lengthen without tearing.

Inside your joints the bone ends are covered with a smooth, shiny, white material called articular cartilage. When healthy joints move, the smooth bone ends glide across each other, constantly oiled by the small amounts of fluid within each joint. The health and integrity of articular cartilage is primarily dependent upon frequent movements of joints and the availability of full ranges of joint movement. Also, unless they are regularly stretched in all directions, joints tend to stiffen with age and only maintain the amount of movement that you use regularly. This is one reason why dancers and gymnasts spend so much time with their stretching routines every day. Imagine suddenly having to do the "splits" if you were stiff.

Stretching muscles is essential for adolescents during growth spurts and becomes more and more important over the age of thirty, so it is a good idea to make this part of your daily practice routine from day one. When young people grow, their bones grow first and then their muscles catch up. When they have been left behind in length, stretching muscles helps to protect them from strains and micro tears with strong use. By the age of thirty, most muscles are beginning to change yet again. They become increasingly less elastic and the ones you use a lot become shorter and more powerful. This is how imbalances lead to faulty positioning of the arm bone in the shoulder. To counteract this, it is necessary to stretch the strong shoulder muscles regularly, particularly before and after playing. Muscles tighten up and shorten with effort, so it is very important to stretch them again after practicing or playing hard.

Muscles should be stretched slowly and gently. Never bounce. Never cause the slightest pain or discomfort. All you should feel as you stretch is the sensation of stiffness or tightness in the muscle slowly lessening, and you will find you can move a little further into the stretch position. Research indicates that most muscles need about 30 seconds of stretching to lengthen appreciably. A little more length can be gained by maintaining a stretch for up to 60 seconds. Muscle stretches should be repeated three to four times each, for maximum effectiveness.

Cool Downs

After strenuous activity, repeat your warm-up exercises and stretches to avoid athletic muscle aches, just as sprinters will continue to jog or walk for a while after their race, then stretch carefully when back in the dressing room. This is far more effective and independent than being massaged after hard work.

Stretching and Strengthening Exercises

Shoulder Joint Flexibility Stretches

1) Find something you can hold onto at about waist height, e.g., the kitchen sink or a railing. Bend forward from the hips, keeping your back, neck and arms straight, until your body is lower than your hands and you can feel the stretch in your shoulder joints. Stay there 5 to 10 seconds, to give the joints a good stretch. If you are tall enough to reach the top of a door frame, you can do this joint stretch by taking a small step through the doorway while your hands press against the top of the other side of the door frame.

2) Rotation stretches for the shoulder joints can be done in several ways. On the floor, lying on your back, place your hands behind your neck so that you are lying as if sunbathing. Your arms should be resting comfortably on the floor. When drying your back after a shower, use the towel to pull your hand up your back to at least the height of your shoulder blades. If you are very flexible, you will be able to touch your hands (see photo 33, p. 113).

Pectoral Muscle Stretches: Fig. 17, p. 114

All you need for equipment is an open doorway. The stretches are done with your hands at three different heights:

      a. as high as you can comfortably reach
      b. at shoulder level
      c. at hip level

Step through the doorway with one foot and lean through, chest leading, like a ship's figurehead. Lean through just until you feel resistance in your pectoral (chest) muscles. Stop at that point and wait 30 seconds until you feel the muscle's resistance disappear as it lengthens in response to the gentle, insistent stretching. Repeat each stretch three times, just taking off the pressure, briefly, between each stretch. Then stretch the deltoid muscle.

Deltoid Muscle Stretches: Fig. 18, p. 114

Stand upright, with good posture. Put your right arm behind your back, until the back of your right hand rests against your left buttock. Grasp your right wrist with your left hand. Let your right arm relax and feel limp, while your left hand stretches it, pulling down gently towards the back of your left leg. If you lean slightly to your left at the same time, you will feel the right arm being

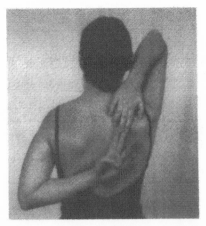

Photo 33. Shoulders' rotation stretch showing very good flexibility.

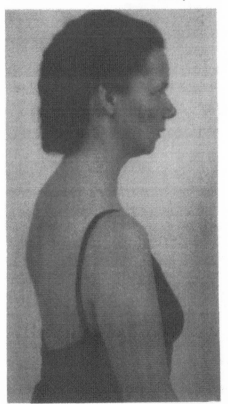
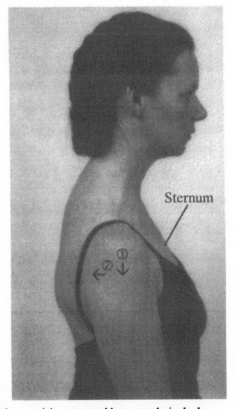

Photo 34. How to correct the faulty shoulder position caused by muscle imbalance. The shoulder, left, is positioned too high and too far forward in the socket. The shoulder, right, is repositioned correctly, by pulling the humerus downward, ① and backward, ② in the joint. The sternum, chest bone, has also been lifted.

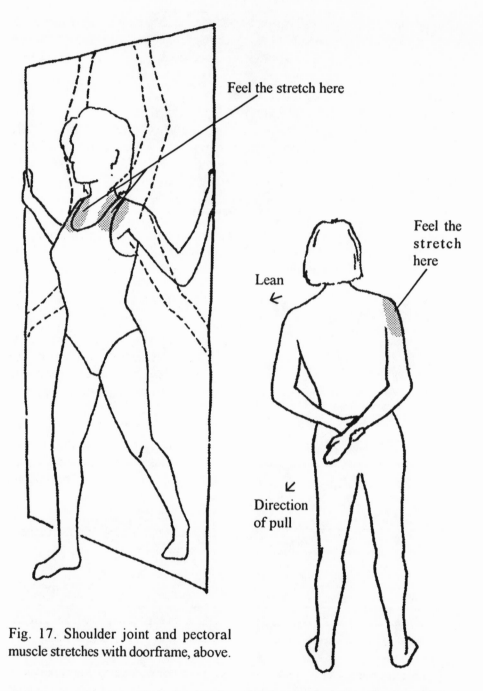

Feel the stretch here

Lean

Feel the stretch here

Direction of pull

Fig. 17. Shoulder joint and pectoral muscle stretches with doorframe, above.

Fig. 18. Deltoid muscle stretch.

pulled downward in the shoulder joint and the deltoid muscle being stretched. It must not hurt to do this. Again, hold the stretch for about 30 seconds, until you feel the tightness in the arm relax. Repeat three times. Repeat with the other arm.

Strengthening Exercises for Shoulders

Strengthening exercises for shoulders are very precise and need to be initially practiced in front of a mirror to ensure you are in the correct starting position:

a. Stand facing a mirror, maintaining excellent posture.
b. Hold a piece of elastic or a 15 lb. (7 kg) spring with handles between your hands, with your elbows bent 90 degrees.
c. Lift your chest bone, the sternum, so that your shoulders drop backward a little and are relaxed. The "horizon" of your shoulders, between your neck and the points of your shoulders, should be level and equally relaxed.
d. Look at your upper arms. Imagine the ball at the top of each one, in the shoulder joint, and pull each ball down half an inch (1cm) in the socket.

You should see very little movement in the mirror. One way to get the feel of this small, important movement is to push your elbows half an inch (1cm) toward the floor. Relax, then practice this a few times until you can see the movement in your mind's eye as well as feel it happening inside the shoulder joint (see photo 34, p. 113).

Meanwhile watch yourself carefully in the mirror to be sure you are not being over-vigorous and moving the whole shoulder area up and down. Very little should be seen to move, but you have corrected any tendency toward your arms becoming positioned too high in the shoulder joints because of all the playing you have already done.

e. Now, having first pulled the balls down in the sockets, pull them one quarter of an inch (6mm) backward in the sockets.

Again, very little movement should be seen in the mirror. Practice this until you can easily do both movements downward and backward, in succession. You are now able to correct the forward pull of your strong pectoral muscles and the upward pull of the deltoid muscle. Practice this often – no one will notice!

f. Maintaining this corrected shoulder joint position, keep your elbows held tightly against your sides and stretch the elastic held between your hands, slowly. Slowly return to the starting position and relax (see photo 44, p. 116).

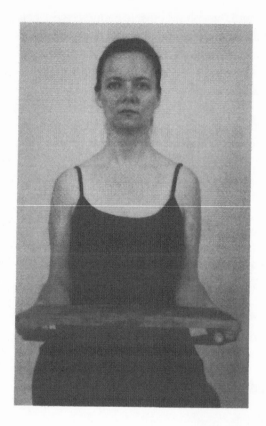

Note that the shoulder joints are correctly positioned and the elbows are held against the body.

Showing the development of muscle bulk on the shoulder blades as a result of practicing this exerceise

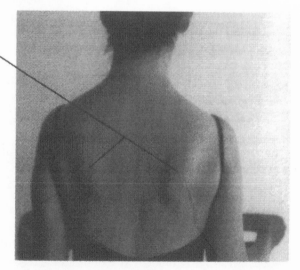

Photo 35. Strengthening exercises for the shoulder's rotator cuff muscles using elastic resistance.

If you have mastered this technique it will be a pain-free exercise and anyone watching your shoulder blades from behind will see the muscles on the lower two-thirds of each shoulder blade expanding and contracting with effort. This is how to strengthen those important rotator cuff muscles, infra spinatus and teres minor.

Note: Help is available if you cannot figure this exercise out. A physiotherapist can use a small muscle stimulator as a teaching device. This has small electrodes which can be used to make your infraspinatus and teres minor muscles contract then relax. You learn to join in, until you can do this exercise without help from the machine. Similarly, a bio-feedback machine can be used to show you how strongly and precisely you can isolate and contract those muscles.

Exercise Prescription for Shoulder Strengthening

Start off with five repetitions, three times a day. Increase over a month until you can do 100 repetitions spread over the day. Be patient, build up repetitions slowly.

If you are playing long hours, you may need to do even more. If you are resting, you may slacken off a bit, but strengthen up again before you start anything strenuous. Build this exercise into your daily life. Try doing it at every stoplight when you are driving, by sitting straight, repositioning the shoulder joints downward and backward and trying to pull the steering wheel apart. (Should you succeed, you have gone too far!)

Caution!

If you have any pain while doing this exercise *it is essential that you stop immediately.* Remember pain weakens the muscles you are trying to strengthen. Go and find an orthopedic physiotherapist because you may already have a shoulder impingement injury and need individual attention. On the other hand, you may just need some one-on-one tuition to get this complicated exercise exactly right, then you can continue training on your own.

Carry the elastic or spring with you everywhere. As you get stronger you may need to increase the strength of the resistance, but there is no need to make it a very heavy, difficult exercise to do. You are training these little muscles for endurance as much as brute strength, so the number of repetitions done correctly is just as important as the amount of resistance you use.

One habit which may need correcting is sleeping with your arms above your head, in the so-called "impingement position." You may need to tie your arms down for a while, if this is a long-established sleeping position. Just do your best to break this habit. Lying prone or face down on a firm bed, with your arms above your head can also create pressure on the inside of your elbow joints, where the nerves run through a groove, around the "funny bones" toward their destinations in the hands. Hence, you can awake with numb fourth and fifth fingers and imagine all sorts of nonexistent injuries.

Elbows

Elbows do not like to be stretched, so leave them alone. If you cannot fully bend and stretch your elbows or turn your hands palms up and palms down because of pain or injury, you need professional help and advice.

Wrists

Wrist joints usually like to be stretched backward (extension). Stretching your wrist joints forward (flexion), so that the palms of your hands move toward the front of your forearms is poorly tolerated. In fact, this stretch done with the elbows kept straight is a test for two common playing injuries, carpel tunnel syndrome and lateral epicondylitis (tennis elbow). Should you feel any discomfort at the elbow or any other odd sensation in your hands while trying this stretch, report this to your physiotherapist. Check this stretch briefly, but do not overdo it (unless you are following a physiotherapy exercise prescription after an injury).

Fingers

Finger joints usually like to be fully bent and stretched, with a little overpressure administered to each one in turn by the other hand (see fig. 22, p 124.) Stretching the fingers wide apart and together again also prepares them for action. Do not force this movement artificially. Simply allow the hands to stretch as far as they can, without help.

Forearm Muscles

Stretching the forearm muscles that work the hardest for musicians means stretching the muscles that come from the inside of the elbow and from the front of the forearm. Above the wrist, they change into tendons that you can see in the front of your wrist if you make a fist. These tendons bend your fingers and provide them with the power to press keys, pluck strings and hold mallets, etc. To stretch these strong flexor muscles, the elbow must be straight and the wrist and fingers extended (bent backward). Have the arm either hanging down in front of you or resting on a table as you use your other hand to apply the stretch by pulling the wrist and fingers gently backward (see photo 36, p. 119).

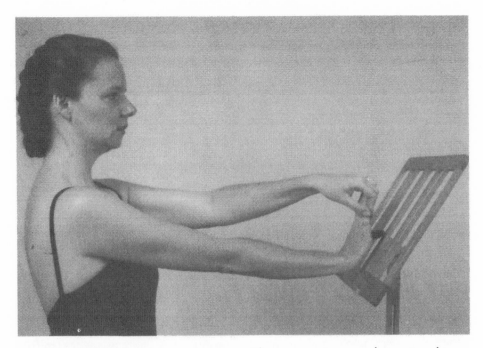

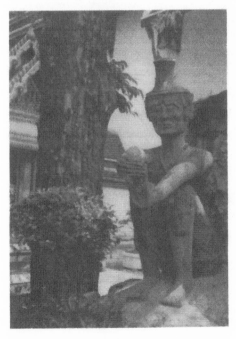

Above, onstage wrist extension position to stretch the forearm muscle used for playing. Left, an ancient statue in Bangkok's Wat Po temple, demonstrating the same stretch.

Photo 36. Wrist extension and forearm muscles stretch.

Some pianists stretch both arms at once by sitting on their hands palms down, but it all depends on the length of your arms. As you can see in the bottom left photo on page 119, this exercise has been performed for centuries as depicted by the statue in Bangkok, reputed to be over 2,000 years old.

Give these muscles the full 30-second stretch, repeated three times, after initial warm-ups and as part of your cool-down.

Strengthening Exercises

Strengthening exercises for the arms and hands of musicians are unnecessary and often cause trouble. Simply play. If you compare the strength of your grip with that of a nonmusican friend of similar sex and build using a grip dynamometer, any concerns you may have should quickly evaporate. (Unless, of course, your friend is a secret bodybuilder.)

Spinal Stretches and Exercises

A healthy spine needs to have full, pain-free movements in all its available directions. Regaining spinal movements may give you "exercise aches" at first. These should resolve rapidly as you get used to the new activity. Stretches and exercises should not increase any existing aches and pains.

Neck and Back Flexion: Forward Bending

Because of our lifestyles, we seldom lose the ability to bend our necks or backs forward (flexion). You can test neck flexion by touching your chin to your chest and back flexion by lying on your back and hugging both knees to your chest. Most people can bend forward to reach beyond their knees. Being able to touch your toes or even place your hands on the floor between your feet indicates that you have long hamstring muscles in the backs of your thighs. It is not a good exercise. It is okay to check these stretches occasionally, but we are always bending in that direction and these are overused movements. Do not practice them repeatedly or very often.

Neck and Back Rotation: Twisting

Similarly, if you drive, you are unlikely to lose the ability to turn your head and look over your shoulder either way. Twisting stretches for the neck and low back should be checked occasionally to ensure you still have those movements, but it is not a good idea to practice them repeatedly as exercises, because repeated or sustained twisting movements are stressful for your spinal discs.

Sideways Bending

Sideways bending of the neck or back can be given an occasional stretch to check you can still do this, but does not need practicing. People who keep their neck bent sideways to hold the telephone, for example, often develop arm or hand tingling or pain as a result. Musicians who play with their heads tilted over to one side get into similar trouble. Sideways bending is a movement used to diagnose neck and back problems rather than a beneficial exercise or stretch.

Neck Retraction: Chicken Exercise. Fig. 19, p. 122.

One movement that we do lose in the neck is called *retraction* or backward gliding. It is the opposite movement to poking your chin forward in a pugnacious manner. To check neck retraction, start with good posture, then try drawing your head back on your shoulders as if withdrawing from an obnoxious smell. You should be able to move your head far enough back on the shoulders to make two or three double chins and, briefly, be unable to breathe or swallow. Obviously you do not stay in that position! Just go as far as you can, give a little over-pressure with your hand across your jaw or mouth, and let go immediately. Repeated, slowly and rhythmically five to ten times, this will gradually restore one of the movements most people lose. You should be able to retract your neck until your ears are positioned behind your shoulder joints. Practice this exercise in the car by touching the back of your head to the headrest, which should be at the height of the middle of your head. Ask a child to do this and you will see how much retraction you started out with. It can be regained, but regain it slowly and gently, rather than trying to undo twenty years of accumulated stiffness in one long weekend. If this exercise causes you any lingering neck discomfort or arm symptoms, stop. Consult an orthopedic physiotherapist for individual coaching.

Until you can retract your neck to where your ears are actually behind the level of your shoulder joints, you cannot expect to be able to maintain perfect posture. This is because joints hate to stay right at the far end of their available movement range. If you can only retract your head to mid-position, i.e., until your ears are directly above the point of your shoulder, your head will soon inevitably move forward until you are once again in your old, familiar, head-poking forward position. Don't despair! With practice and very gentle over-pressures, you will gradually regain more movement.

You will also notice that your neck will appear to have lengthened and that you are suddenly looking taller and more impressive. Long-standing TMJ (tempero-mandibular, or jaw joint) pain problems frequently clear up once the head is again balanced correctly upon the neck, instead of constantly poking ahead of the rest of the body.

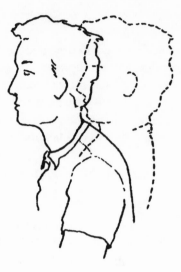

Fig. 19. Neck retraction (chicken exercise).

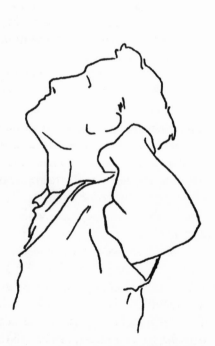

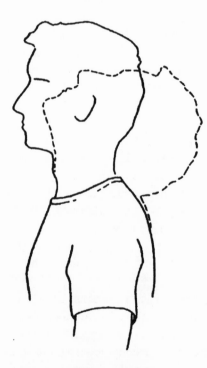

Fig. 20. Neck extension with hands
supporting the neck.

Fig. 21. Neck extension
without support.

Neck Extension: Bending Backward. Figs. 20 & 21, p. 122

Testing backward bending or extension of the neck and back is a true test of spinal flexibility, because these are movements that most musicians do not use and therefore lose. Start by sitting or standing with perfect posture. Now retract your head and neck backward as far as you can, without applying over-pressure. Next, lift up your chin and bend your head backward to look at the ceiling. Go as far as you can. Full neck movement and flexibility is when you can comfortably rest the back of your head on your upper back. If you have not looked up like this for years, you may find this difficult to do. Sometimes holding your neck with both hands, using the hands to lift the weight of your head upright again, makes it easier.

The only times most people look up is at an air show or when painting the ceiling. If you have stiffened up, it can be very uncomfortable attempting to move this way again. This is why many exercise classes avoid this exercise and believe it is a movement to avoid. On the contrary, it is a movement that is essential for a healthy, happy, pain-free neck.

Any significant dizziness, loss of balance, increasing neck or arm pain or other strange symptoms means *stop!* Find an orthopedic physiotherapist for individual teaching. Most young necks really like this exercise as soon as they try it. Many older necks are very stiff and have great difficulty regaining this movement if they have avoided it for years. Get help if you need it.

Once you can extend your neck fully and comfortably, healthy people can give their neck a beneficial stretch by hanging backward over the edge of the bed or coffee table, as children hang from jungle gyms (see photo 37, p. 124). Agile young musicians can even manage this using a sturdy chair. (This has to be seen to be believed and you can try it at your own risk.) Neck retraction and neck extension exercises are also a powerful antidote to the tendency some older musicians have to gradually stiffen into a stooped posture. Grandmother was right yet again . . . exercise is good for you.

Low Back Extensions: Bending Backward

Full backward flexibility or extension of the low back is tested by lying on your stomach, then pushing only your upper body off the floor by straightening your arms. If you have full extension flexibility your pelvis and hip bones will stay on the floor. Again, children do this effortlessly and most adults lose this movement unless they practice yoga or gymnastics (see photo 38, p. 125). Full extension can eventually be regained if you do this as a daily stretch. Avoid overexuberance and do the exercise gently, or you will make your back hurt. All stiff movements should be gently coaxed back to normal, never bullied.

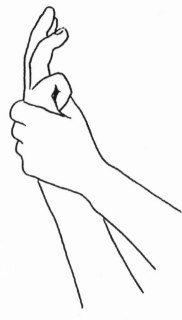

Fig. 22. Fully bend and fully stretch all finger joints with brief gentle overpressure.

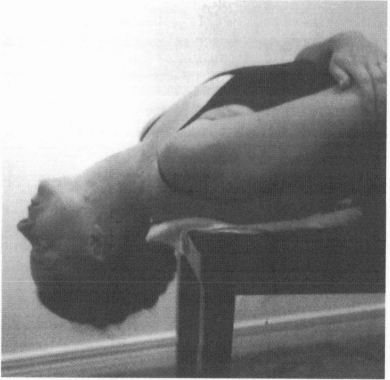

Photo 37. A good stretch for healthy, flexible necks.

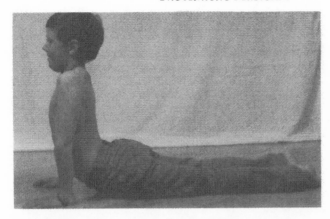

This is full spinal extension and it tests the low back's flexibility. Note the position of the arms.

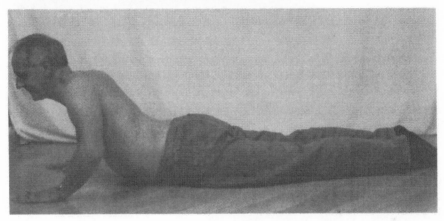

Adults lose their ability, above, to do this beneficial movement . . .

. . . but can regain it over time, right, through gentle persistant exercise.

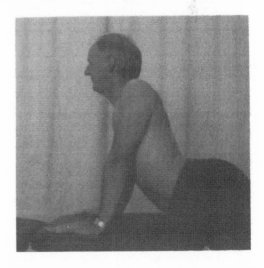

Photo 38. Father and son team demonstrating back extension flexibility. Shown at different stages of life.

Back extension exercises can be done throughout the day by simply putting your hands on the low back and leaning backward over them, briefly. Repeat this rocking movement five to ten times. It is known as the "wise farmer's back bend" and should be repeated many times throughout the day to counteract the effects of sitting and forward bending (fig. 23, p. 127).

Sit-ups

Never do sit-ups in any shape or form (see fig. 24, p. 127). This is an ill-conceived exercise, designed in response to the mistaken belief that sit-ups efficiently strengthen the abdominal muscles which, in turn, will protect your back from injury. Repeated sit-ups squeeze the front of your spinal discs until they bulge out at the back, precisely the scenario you need to avoid. Repeated sit-ups frequently are responsible for neck and back pain. Cats, dogs and other vertebrates would never dream of doing such a bizarre exercise to keep fit. Instead, they stretch their spines into an extension curve before running around.

There is no particular reason to have abnormally strong abdominal muscles, unless you are a boxer, regularly fielding blows to the torso. Very strong people hurt their backs just as easily as anyone else if they do not maintain a lordosis while lifting, or if they work bent over or sit slouched. Many people who suddenly become concerned about the shape of their enlarging abdomens would do better to lose a little superfluous weight than to try to strengthen the buried muscles.

If you really insist in pursuing this goal, your abdominal muscles should be strengthened in the upright position. Wear a backpack and climb up and down hills or a ravine. Your abdominal muscles work hardest when holding you upright and will have to work even harder to counteract the weight pulling you backward. Giving children a piggyback ride (not on your shoulders) has the same effect. Carry sufficient weight to feel it pulling you backward, but not so much that you have to walk bent over forward to balance it. Backpacks with a frame are the most comfortable and allow you to stand and walk upright, where your spine is safe. Walking and running, even without a backpack, keep your abdominal muscles working and as strong as you need them for normal activities of daily life. If they did not work hard, you would fall over backward with every step forward!

Leg Stretches: Calf Muscles. Fig. 25, p. 128

1) To stretch your calf muscles, stand facing a wall, or rail, or the kitchen sink and rest your hands on them for balance. (There is no need to lean heavily or try to push the wall down.) Stand up straight and have one foot a step ahead of the other one. Point your toes straight forward and bend the front knee slightly.

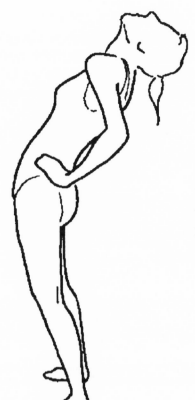

Fig. 23. Wise farmer's back bend stretch. Do this often. Make sure you are bending only your lower back and not at the knees

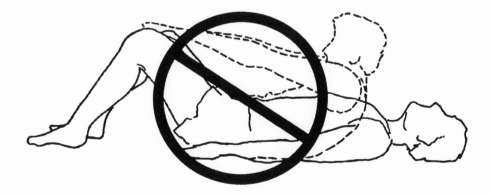

Fig. 24. Sit-ups and curl-ups are NOT recommended exercises.

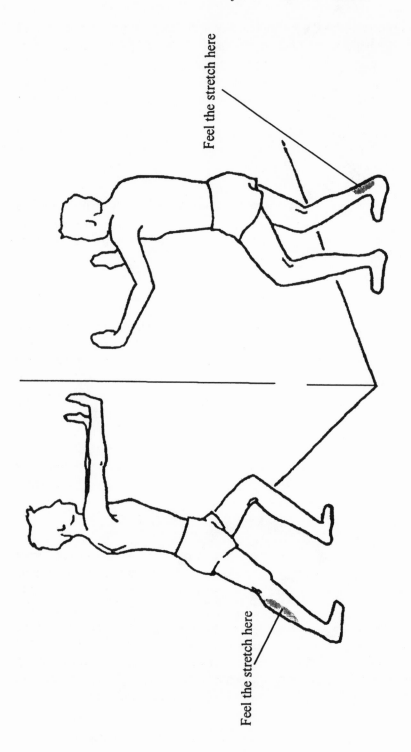

Feel the stretch here

Feel the stretch here

Fig. 26. Achilles' tendon stretch.

Fig. 25. Calf muscle stretch.

Keeping your heels on the floor, slowly move your hips forward toward the wall until you feel a gentle stretch in the calf muscle of the straight back leg. Be sure that your heel stays on the ground and that your toes still point forward. Hold this for 30 to 60 seconds or until you feel the tightness in the muscle disappear, as the calf muscle lengthens. Repeat this with the other leg. Try three repetitions of 30 seconds for each leg.

2) To stretch the calf muscle tendon (Achilles' tendon) start in the same position, but slowly bend the back knee as well, just slightly, until you feel some tightness in the back leg, just above the ankle (see fig. 26, p. 128). Check to see that your toes are still pointing straight forward and keep both heels firmly planted on the floor. Hold this for 30 to 60 seconds until the slight tightness in the tendon disappears. This tendon needs very gentle stretching, so don't do this stretch forcefully. Sudden, forceful stretches can tear very strong muscles and tendons. Try three repetitions of 30 seconds for each leg.

Quadriceps Muscle: Front of Thigh. Fig. 27, p. 130

Stand facing a wall, railing or anything firm that you can hold to maintain your balance. Stand on one leg. Bend the other knee behind you and take hold of the foot in the opposite hand. Stand straight, with good posture and with your knees on the same level – not one in front of the other. Now gently pull the foot you have hold of toward the opposite buttock, so that your knee is bending at its normal angle. Pull gently until you feel some tightness in the front of the thigh. Hold this 30 to 60 seconds or until you feel the slight tightness disappear as your quadriceps lengthen. Repeat with the other leg. If you are very flexible, you may have to take the flexed knee further back, behind the level of the leg you are standing on, to feel a stretch. Try three repetitions of 30 seconds for each leg.

Hamstring Muscle: Back of Thigh. Fig. 28, p. 130

This stretch is frequently performed incorrectly. You should keep your head up and your back straight or slightly arched throughout the stretch. Stand facing a flight of stairs. Put one heel onto the highest stair you can comfortably reach while keeping both legs straight and an upright posture without strain. Clasp your hands together loosely behind your back. Now slowly push your chest forward, *without bending your low back*. It will just take a small amount of movement before you feel tension in the back of the thigh of your raised leg. Stay in that position 20 to 60 seconds or until the tightness disappears. Repeat with the other leg. Try three repetitions of 30 seconds for each leg.

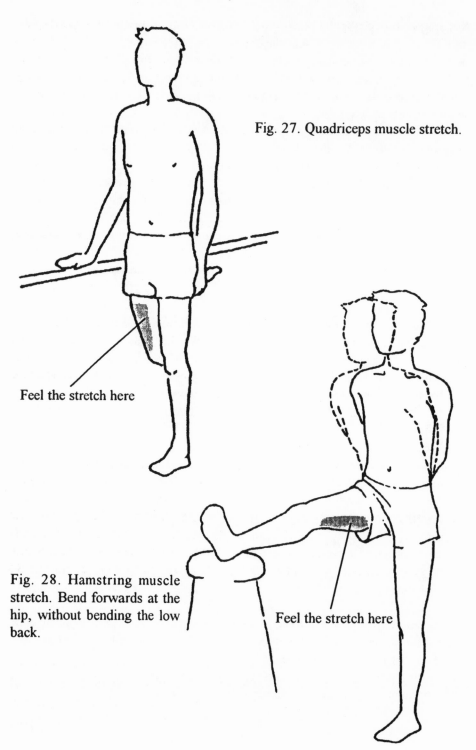

Fig. 27. Quadriceps muscle stretch.

Feel the stretch here

Fig. 28. Hamstring muscle stretch. Bend forwards at the hip, without bending the low back.

Feel the stretch here

Hip Adductor Muscles: Inside of Thighs and Groin. Fig. 29, p. 132

Sit with good posture, close to a wall for support. Put the soles of your feet together, with your heels as close to your body as you can put them comfortably. Now allow your knees to sink towards the floor, until you feel a gentle stretch in the groin area and the inside of your thighs. Maintaining this position for 30 to 60 seconds will allow the weight of your legs to maintain this stretch. There is no need to push the knees down with your hands unless you cannot feel any tightness without doing that. Try three repetitions of 30 seconds each.

Hip Abductor Muscles: Outside of Hip and Thigh. Fig. 30, p. 132

Stand with your right leg crossed over behind the left leg. Without bending forward at all, lean your body over to the left until you feel tightness down the outside of your right hip and thigh. This is a difficult position to maintain for the required 30 to 60 seconds. If you prefer, you can do it lying on a table or on the edge of your bed. Turn the diagram sideways and you'll see how you could lie on your left side, with your back close to the edge of the table or bed, then let the right leg hang off the bed behind you to feel the stretch. If you do it this way, make sure you don't twist your body (or fall off the table!). Keep the side of your hip pointing up toward the ceiling the whole time. Again, repeat this with the other leg. Try three repetitions of 30 to 60 seconds, each leg.

Piriformis Muscles: Deep Hip Muscle. Fig. 31, p. 132

Sit on the floor with your left leg straight out in front of you. Bend your right leg and cross it over the left leg until your right foot is on the floor by the outside of your left knee. Either hug the right knee, or hold it in place using your left arm, as shown. Now turn your body gently toward the right, until you feel tightness deep inside the right buttock, almost exactly where your weight is going through your seat. Hold this stretch for 30 to 60 seconds or until that deep, tight feeling disappears. Repeat with the other leg. Try three repetitions of 30 seconds for each leg.

Sports, Fitness, and Cross Training

These important subjects are frequently either neglected by musicians or pursued with more vigor than benefit. In order to withstand the physical strains and stresses of prolonged playing, musicians should aim to become very physically fit. You do not need excessive strength to play an instrument for several hours,

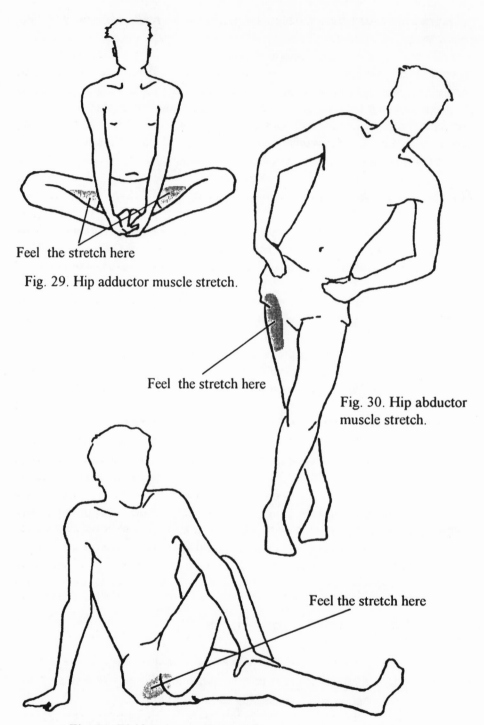

Feel the stretch here

Fig. 29. Hip adductor muscle stretch.

Feel the stretch here

Fig. 30. Hip abductor
muscle stretch.

Feel the stretch here

Fig. 31. Piriformis muscle stretch.

but you do need good general health, including a healthy cardiovascular system, above-average conditioning and remarkable endurance. Fit people do not tire as quickly, and can concentrate and maintain a good sitting posture longer.

Learning from athletes, your physical activities should be tailored to fit your needs, so look for aerobic activities rather than weight lifting or over-strenuous upper body work. For general conditioning and increased fitness, exercise the large muscles of your legs. Skating, cycling, in-line skating, running, dancing (but not the twist), backpacking and walking up and down hills are all excellent cross-training activities that will improve your cardiovascular fitness level and general conditioning. Swimming keeps people very fit, too, but if playing involves holding your arms away from your side most of the time, avoid overhead strokes or you may overstrengthen shoulder muscles to the point of causing an impingement syndrome. Breast stroke, side stroke and back stroke, sculling with arms down by your side, are fine. Most musicians should avoid upper body workouts, as the majority of your injuries are due to overworked muscles. It just does not make sense to make the same playing muscles work even harder and longer. Also, you increase the likelihood of causing serious muscle imbalances around the shoulder if you lift weights to develop your pectoral, deltoid, biceps, triceps and latissimus dorsi muscles.

Gym Work

If you belong to a gym or fitness club, it is best to stay away from their machines that work the arms, neck and low back. Several musicians with playing injuries have told me how much they enjoy building well-defined muscles in their arms, shoulders and torso and that they want to look good. Unfortunately, it is just not worth it. If you were planning a career as a stand-in for Tarzan, swinging through the jungle on vines, all the excess bulk would probably be put to good use – but you are a musician. Brute strength and shortened, bulky biceps glistening with baby oil just do not help your career in any way. In fact quite the opposite (and anyway, have you ever heard Tarzan play the violin?).

You are, however, safe using the leg machines. Exercycles, stair climbers, treadmills, lying down leg-press machines, hip abductor and adductor machines and "legs only" ski machines are all fine. Rowing machines are not. Make sure you warm up, cool down and stretch your leg muscles before and after using the machines, especially if you are over 30 years old, to avoid muscle tears.

Gym Classes

Gym classes can be fun. Aerobic classes and step classes give a good workout and are safe as long as you avoid pain, stop before you get too weary and remember to monitor your pulse, staying within your target heart rate zone. There should be charts displayed in your gym to show you how to do this. Ask for assistance if this is new to you. Remember, you are an athlete.

Here is a word of warning about gym and exercise classes. In general, I find most of them still put too much emphasis on forward bending movements, such as touching your toes or sitting on the floor and reaching over to touch your feet, pulling your head down to touch your knees. This is because most instructors have been taught that these forward movements increase spinal flexibility. As you now know, if you have read the previous chapter on the spine, this is incorrect information. The beneficial flexibility we lose is the ability to bend backward, not forward. It is often easier to just substitute backward stretches for your back and neck for the instructor's forward stretches. Also, do not do "pelvic tilt" exercises, which are still in vogue in many gyms.

Sports

Tennis, baseball, golf, volleyball and squash regularly produce overuse injuries in the shoulder, arms and wrists. Tennis elbows, golfers' elbows, volleyball thumbs, fingers, and forearms, as well as baseball, swimming, tennis and squash shoulders, are all regularly brought in for care and repair in our Sports Injuries Clinic. Try soccer instead, if you like team sport, then bowling or curling, but do not sweep. Cross-country skiing is a great sport for musicians, using the legs strongly and very little pole work. Horseback riding is highly recommended, especially English style, which promotes excellent posture for the head, neck and back to balance the horse. Dressage riders learn to push the back of their neck backward to touch their jacket collar – exactly the exercise we use to promote perfect head posture when driving or playing. The rider's elbows are tucked in and a well-mannered horse does not require the reins to be used with any force. Sitting on a horse is a very good position for your low back too, with your knees lower than your hips and some weight going through your feet as well as your seat (see fig. 11, p. 60).

However, if your idea of riding is barrel racing, broncobusting or taming a maverick mustang by wrestling it to the ground, please remove riding from my list of recommended sports for musicians. Poorly trained horses can hurt your wrists and arms if they are determined to demonstrate their obviously superior strength. They can also break your neck, so choose your riding establishment with care.

Hobbies and Other Activities

When you consider that most neck and back problems are due to poor posture and too much bending and sitting, it makes sense to examine your favorite hobbies and leisure pursuits from an ergonomic point of view.

If, as a musician, you spend many hours sitting still or driving with your head slightly forward, these are positions to avoid whenever possible when you are not performing, practicing or traveling. This does not mean you cannot play chess, knit, read or collect stamps, but it does mean that you may need to interrupt these activities often or change the position you use. For "static" hobbies, learn to use less stressful positions, e.g., lying or standing, rather than sitting. Take the weight of your head on your hands to ease your neck. Stand or move about more. If you paint or draw, use an easel. Read lying on your front. Interrupt studying, writing or typing occasionally. If you run up and down stairs a few times your improved circulation may even help you finish that crossword or essay.

Computers can get you into trouble. Operators arrive frequently for treatment, with wrist, neck and back problems, so use them cautiously, with a good set-up and many breaks. Stay away from them if you already have playing injuries. "Other work" is hardly a hobby, but is often a fact of life for students to survive and eat. Students are already prone to developing playing injuries because of their escalating hours of practice. Add to this a job that is very heavy or strenuous for the upper body and arms, and your body can get into trouble with overuse symptoms and serious muscle imbalances. Actors, dancers and singers can survive a waiter's job, but it is a bad choice for musicians. I realize that it is hard to pick and choose when money is in short supply, but if there is any choice at all then aim for a job requiring leg work, such as delivering flyers, a cycling courier, helping in a summer camp or being a lifeguard, anything that keeps you up and moving without carrying heavy weights.

Summary of Daily Exercise Routines

I. General Conditioning Protocol

Daily if playing regularly, alternate days if playing occasionally:
  a. Warm-up   5 minutes
  b. Stretch   Calf muscles - 30 seconds, 3 times each leg
                Hamstrings   - 30 seconds, 3 times each leg
                Quadriceps   - 30 seconds, 3 times each leg
                Neck retractions and extensions - 10 times
                Back extensions - 10 times

    c. Cross training
       Cycle, in-line skate, run/walk briskly, leg machines, stair climber, ice
       skate, dance etc. - 20 to 30 minutes of leg work
    d. Cool-down - 5 minutes
    e. Stretch - redo all stretches faithfully, to prevent muscle exercise aches.
    f. Ice pack any sore muscles for 10 to 15 minutes, until red. (Use a cold,
       wet cloth between your skin and a soft ice pack, or stroke the muscle
       repeatedly with a wet ice cube.)

II. Strengthening Rotator Cuff Muscles - Daily

    a. Use mirror.
    b. Correct posture.
    c. Position the head of the armbone (humerus) down and backward in
       the socket.
    d. Bend your elbows to 90 degrees and tuck them firmly against your
       ribs.
    e. Loop the elastic around your wrists.
    f. Pull your hands away from each other, slowly, as if opening double
       doors, stretching the elastic.
    g. Hold briefly, then slowly return.
    h. Repeat 5 times.

Do several sessions daily. Increase repetitions gradually working up to 100 times daily. The more you play, the more of these you need to do.

Relaxation and Mental Imaging

These are two acquired skills which improve with regular practice. Both are of great value and assist your mind and body to survive physically and mentally stressful careers. A skillful relaxation tutor will teach you more than the time-honored total body relaxation techniques that require a peaceful, quiet place to lie down. Advanced training can teach you how to relax while sitting (without falling off your chair) and, among other useful skills, how to relax despite noise and seeming chaos all around you. Practicing relaxation helps to lower rising blood pressure for tense people and has many other pleasing effects. It releases "endorphins," the body's natural drug, which promotes a feeling of well-being similar to a runner's "high." Once you have been taught how to relax using methods which are particularly suited to you and your lifestyle, you should be able to practice this independently and benefit from the results whenever your stress level needs attention.

Mental Practice

Mental practice or visualization is nothing new to professional athletes, but is still relatively unknown among musicians. It is not the same thing as thinking about music. In order to understand its use and value, one needs first to consider how the brain learns new skills, including music, and how it perfects performing these skills and retains them for future use. A few examples might help. If you remember how overwhelmed you were by your first driving lesson and how exhausted you felt at the end of that hour, you will probably appreciate how much energy the brain uses to learn a new skill. For most people, it takes many lessons before they can appreciate the scenery as well as drive – the concentration needed to steer, change gears and indicate turns all at once is, at first, all consuming. However, little by little the brain accumulates these actions and when to use which, and moves them to another area of the brain for storage and instant retrieval. This area requires far less energy to use and eventually one is able to drive through complex traffic situations without consciously considering the physical steps involved. The brain is functioning on automatic and the right things happen *IF and ONLY IF* the correct information has been stored there in the first place. The brain stores physical skills just as a computer stores data. If you fill it with faulty information, that is what it will give you back again whenever it is running on automatic. What a tremendous responsibility that places upon teachers and coaches and how much weight that gives to their advice to "get it right the first time." You may have noticed how few self-taught, two-finger typists ever learn to use all their fingers on a keyboard.

Mental imaging or visualization is a very useful technique which speeds up the process of moving a newly learned physical skill from the exhausting area of the brain to the storage area, without physically repeating the actions many times. Sufficient data have been collected from competitive athletes and their sports psychologists to provide convincing evidence that mental imaging really works. Study after study shows that athletes who practice mentally as well as physically outperform their competitors who only practice physically. They also improve upon their previous performances, for example, in speed or height and in accuracy. How does it work? No one is quite sure yet. However, it appears that if you can recreate in your imagination the exact sensation of performing a physical skill, your brain will accept this as if you had really done it.

People do this in many ways. Equestrians walking around the jumps before a competition visualize how to tackle the course. Their horse uses new skills at every new jump, but is obviously helped by an experienced rider who has mentally visualized getting both of them over every obstacle beforehand. Public speakers mentally rehearse their "spontaneous" responses to their audiences' questions, often while traveling to assignments, and their performances are enhanced.

When I was growing up, my brother's friend took his father's car keys, started the car and drove it around a corner and into the back of the neighbor's car. I am certain now that this accident would not have happened if he had been able to reach the brake, but he was only two and a half years old at the time. He must have been visualizing how to start and drive the car since before he could walk, by watching adults do it, and probably by mental practicing in his crib at night. The only thing that had held him back before that fateful day was his lack of height. He could not reach the shelf where the keys were kept.

The art of mental practice seems to me to be custom-made for musicians. Most musicians' injuries are overuse injuries, and here is a mental skill which will allow you to replace at least part of your physical practice sessions with brain exercises. Please give it a try.

There are skillful trainers who can teach you many different ways to practice mentally until you find a method that suits you best. I will give you a simple version to try yourself. When you have practiced a piece of music and you have decided exactly how you want it to sound, leave your instrument and either sit, or preferably lie down, in a quiet place. Close your eyes and allow your body to relax and go limp like a rag doll, especially your back, neck, shoulders, arms and hands that need the rest. *In your imagination,* picture yourself returning to the practice room. Close the door behind you and return to your instrument. It is important for successful mental practicing that you use all of your senses, so imagine that you can feel the weight and texture of your instrument and that you can feel the floor under your feet. Smell any familiar, usual fragrances in that room and see the view that you would normally see from the window. Now, in your imagination, resume your practicing. Remember that the performance must be exactly as you wish it to be stored in your brain, so correct any errors in your imaginary playing and practice faultlessly. You should feel as if you are really there, playing and hearing every note. Try short sessions at first. If you find it too difficult to imagine this vividly, find a sports psychologist who is used to exploring other methods of mental practicing with athletes and ask for help. You will doubtless be as surprised as other athletes by your results, and your body's risk of injury is lowered.

Chapter 11

Practicing as an Athletic Musician

Unlike the professional athlete working under the supervision of a multi-dimensional training staff, a musician practices alone. Students, amateurs, orchestral players or soloists will spend a significant portion of their playing time by themselves in a practice room. Lessons with our teachers make up only a small fraction of the total time we spend on the instrument, and teachers themselves are often ill-equipped to serve as our "athletic" coaches. Most music students graduate without having been taught *how* to practice and without any knowledge of functional anatomy, as it relates to playing. To develop safe and effective practice habits, we need to change our approach to our work, thinking like athletes and incorporating principles of sports medicine and psychology.

Pre-Practice Warm - ups

Musicians think of warming up as something they do when they start playing their instruments, but athletes begin their training sessions by warming up before they stretch and perform their sport. Playing *is* our sport, and it is important for us as athletes to warm up and stretch before playing. (See Chapter 10.)

There are countless ways to warm up before playing if you are at home. You could plan your practice session to follow your favorite aerobic activity (cycling, in-line skating, country line dancing, etc.). If you want to kill two birds with one stone, you could vacuum, wash a window or walk your dog to warm up. It takes less than five minutes of arm swings to increase the blood flow to your arms and hands, but if you are feeling lazy you can take a long, hot shower instead.

Pre-Practice Stretches

How many other habits can you develop that will be as quick, easy, cheap and pleasurable as stretching before and after you play? Ideally, you should go through a complete body stretching routine daily. (See Chapter 10.) Just as you would not think of jogging without first doing leg stretches, make sure that before

139

you play you go through a routine that will stretch out at least the upper body muscles that you will be using. Referring to Chapter 10, select stretches for shoulders, arms, wrists and hands as appropriate to your instrument. For instance, anyone playing with their arms up and away from their body could go through the following routine:

    a. Overhead shoulder stretch - 30 seconds, 3 times each side
    b. Deltoid stretch - 30 seconds, 3 times each side
    c. Doorway stretch - 30 seconds, 3 times
    d. Wrist flexion stretch - check briefly
    e. Wrist extension stretch - 30 seconds, 3 times each side

Regardless of your instrument, you probably spend so much time in a head forward position (reading, driving, etc.) that you should incorporate:

    f. Neck retraction and extension exercises - 10 times

If you sit to practice, or play the double-bass, you should also plan on:

    g. Back extension stretches - 10 times

Warming Up on the Instrument

Now that you've warmed up away from the instrument and stretched, it's time for the traditional musician's warm-up with the instrument. In athletic terms, this part of your training session should start off with playing that gets you moving gently, gradually building in intensity, just as Olympic sprinters would start their workout with slow jogging and moderate running before attempting to set a new time on their 100-meter dash. Make sure your body is warm enough. If necessary, turn up the thermostat or wear fingerless gloves.

Some musicians go through a very prescribed regimen of technical exercises at this point in their practice, while others like to plunge right into repertoire. Pedagogical debates aside, both styles can work if you keep athletic training principles in mind. Warm-up material should be moderately demanding and varied, and encourage movement in safe positions. This is not the time to barrel through a cadenza, but even traditional warm-up routines can present less obvious dangers. Evaluate your warm-up to see if what you are playing and *how* you are playing it is appropriate for the beginning of your practice session.

Pianists, for example, have traditionally started their practice session with scales. Scales are fine, but playing through all keys in succession at a very fast tempo does not make sense during your warm-up. A slower tempo and alternating scales with arpeggios, for example, would be more suitable for the beginning of a practice session.

You could sight-read in your warm-up. This can take you through short bits of varied repertoire that are not likely to be as technically demanding as the concerto you're working on (or am I the only violinist who doesn't sight-read Paganini?).

String players can use a wider, more relaxed vibrato when they warm up, or work slowly on intonation without vibrato. Violinists and violists should avoid staying up in high positions which put wrists in dangerously flexed positions. (See Chapter 8.) However, relaxed shifting exercises (like Dont op. 35, #7) or scales that take you briefly into flexion and then back to a neutral position would be appropriate. Low-intensity practice doesn't include double-stops, sautillé bowing, or very long sustained notes. Wind players could include long, sustained notes in their warm-up routine as it is not necessary for them to hold their arm up in the air, while moving as little as possible to do so.

You can use warm-up time to play virtually anything you like as long as you remember that your aims are:

> Gentle movement
> Variety
> Moderate speed
> Neutral body positions

Hot and Heavy Practicing

If you were on a computerized step machine or treadmill at the gym, by this point in your program your heart rate would be elevated and you'd be working up a sweat as you hit your first steep hills. When we practice, we also need to work on those "steep hills" and after you have warmed up is the time to do it. If step machines kept us working at the top of those hills all the time, most of us would find ourselves being carried out of the gym on a stretcher. Yet when we practice, we can get so emotionally and intellectually involved in what we're doing that we push ourselves mercilessly in endless repetitions of the most difficult and "dangerous" material. In the absence of flashing lights telling us that we're in a demanding segment of our workout, we need to keep in touch with how we're feeling and be aware of the intensity and risks of what we are doing.

The physical demands of playing vary from situation to situation. Private practicing, as opposed to playing at a lesson or in an orchestra, allows the musician the most control over how, when and what they will play. Theoretically, if your posture and ergonomics are correct, practicing could be free from risk of injury. In actual fact, this almost total control that we have over our practice environment can backfire. For example, musicians left to their own devices when deciding when to practice may find themselves trying to condense several weeks' worth of practicing into a few days. (Many students have discovered the hard way that this doesn't always work.) And despite our best laid plans, circumstances beyond our control can put us in situations where we suddenly have to increase our practice time. Taking breaks when we practice can present a problem too. In a work environment, regular breaks are scheduled for us and in rehearsals there are often many "stoppages in play" that give us an opportunity to take a brief rest. When we practice on our own we are responsible for setting our own limits and scheduling our own breaks. Sometimes we'll feel like taking breaks every five minutes, but at other times practicing can be such an intense experience that we can find ourselves playing nonstop for long periods of time. If you're a musician who can spend hours at a time practicing you may have to set arbitrary time limits, using an alarm clock if necessary.

Breaks between practice sessions are crucial, but incorporating brief "time outs" *during* a practice session can also enable you to work more safely and more productively. A "break" doesn't mean going out for coffee, but it can mean changing your position with the instrument, or putting it down momentarily while you think about what you're doing. Drinking (water!) is a good habit to get into. Leaving a glass of water on a table near you and developing the habit of regular sipping encourages you to change your position momentarily. Using a tape recorder when you practice is another option. Not only does listening to yourself help you to zero in on what you're going to work on next, but operating the machine provides a built-in opportunity to alter your position. Incorporate stretches and exercises into your practice sessions. (See Chapter 12 concerning onstage stretches and exercises.) Rigidly holding yourself in any one position is not a good idea, so move as much as possible. Beware the metronome trap! With the old-style pendulum metronomes one always had a few seconds' break between repetitions to move the weight and wait for the beat to even out. Put your electronic metronome on a table a few feet away from you, rather than on the stand.

While repetition is a necessary part of practicing, mindless repetition belongs on an assembly line and not in the practice studio. It keeps you locked in one position, it's not productive and it repeatedly stresses the same part of your body in exactly the same way. By incorporating mental imaging techniques (Chapter 10) throughout your practice session, you can get better results with fewer repetitions and give your body a brief respite while maintaining your train of thought.

Any playing that puts you into poor posture can lead to injury. (See Chapter 6.) If your posture goes out the window as soon as you get involved in your work, try videotaping a practice session so you can take an objective look at yourself after the fact. If, despite your best efforts, you can't or won't eliminate all bad postural habits when you play, you need to incorporate "time outs" for correction and alternate stretches and ensure that your posture when you are *not* playing is correct.

There are few instruments that one can play in a completely correct position all the time. A double bass player for example, who refused to play anything at the end of the fingerboard because it put his back into dangerous flexion, could have a healthy spine and an ailing bank account. Most instrumental playing necessitates some time spent with backs or wrists flexed or heads slightly rotated. We must be aware of the risks associated with these positions if we are to successfully avoid injuries. Understanding the anatomy involved in carpal tunnel syndrome, for example, is the first step in preventing it. Examining your playing to discover when your flexed wrist position is putting you at risk would be the next step. Then see if there is anything you can do ergonomically to minimize the degree of flexion. For example, pianists might want to investigate seat height to see if they can favorably change the angle of their wrists. A violist with small hands may want to stay away from an instrument with wide, square upper bouts that make you get into flexion sooner rather than later when you shift. Regardless, upper string players will still need to spend time with wrists in flexion in order to play in high positions. In our private practicing we can control the length of time spent up in the stratosphere and incorporate corrective stretches frequently. Providing lots of variety in a practice session makes whatever you're doing safer. Alternate slow and fast practice, concentrate on one hand at a time (where possible), or work on two different registers of an instrument.

Final Stretches

When you've finished practicing, spend a few more minutes with the instrument gradually winding down and cooling off, choosing the same type of material you used in your warm-up. Once the case is shut, go through whichever job-specific stretches you selected for your warm-up and do them again. Stretching *after* playing is even more important than stretching before, and feels great.

How Much Practice Is Too Much?

How you practice and what you practice can influence the amount of time you can safely spend playing an instrument, but this doesn't mean that you can or should play for an unlimited number of hours each day. Because the demands of instruments and repertoire can vary so much, it is difficult to provide rigid guidelines. While it is impossible to come up with hard and fast rules for musicians, studies of keyboard computer operators can give us some clues. See page 89. There will be times in our careers when we will have to spend more time playing than is "sensible." If you can anticipate when your busiest times will be, train by gradually building up your practice time. Amateur musicians are often caught in this trap as they are not always accustomed to playing every day. Trying to cope with the demands of a summer program or hours of chamber music with friends on weekends can be dangerous. Establishing a baseline of regular playing and training for that summer program would put you in a better position to avoid injury.

Convincing injured musicians that they must play less or stop for a while is difficult enough; advising a healthy one to "cut back" is pointless. When you must play too much, do what you can to make it as safe as possible (stretch carefully and often, take regular breaks, ice after long sessions, spend more time on mental practice). There is *never* any reason to abuse oneself with pointless, ineffective practice or to play in pain and risk injury. Rather than planning to stop playing when you start hurting, plan to stop playing when you stop thinking!

Summary of Good Practice Habits

     a. Warm up without the instrument
     b. Stretch
     c. Correct stressful postures
     d. Ensure your instrument is user-friendly! See Chapter 9
     e. Aim for variety
     f. Move
     g. Overuse your brain cells (these don't wear out!)
     h. Pay attention to your body – recognize healthy fatigue and stop before you hurt

Mental Imaging for Musicians

Glenn Gould once said, "I go days – not only days, but weeks – without touching the piano. I've never seen why it's necessary . . . I play best after two weeks or so that I've laid off."[1] Perhaps part of Gould's genius was his innate ability to learn by thinking rather than doing. While many musicians spend time studying scores and thinking about what they are going to play, actually playing in your mind is a different skill and one that can be learned. Athletes of the musical variety can use mental imaging techniques in much the same way as Olympic athletes do, enhancing performance and moderating the length of time spent playing by limiting stressful and unnecessary repetition and ensuring that practice time is spent efficiently. Of course, for the fanatical player, this means they can still play eight hours a day but get twice as much done!

Despite having developed efficient practice habits, I didn't learn the skill of true mental imaging or realize its value until circumstances forced me to work away from the instrument. When I first resumed playing after my injury, the schedule Barbara put me on was very limiting. I started by playing for five minutes a day and it took a long time before I had the endurance to practice for any length of time. I discovered that, even with such short practice sessions and despite feeling hopelessly "out of shape," my playing skills were returning much faster than I could have expected and my playing improved out of proportion to the amount of practicing I was able to do. During the almost 24 hours I had to wait between practice sessions, I had a lot of time to think about what I was going to do. Unlike the years when I was injured and made a deliberate effort *not* to think about playing, now I constantly imagined myself playing and this was my first step in acquiring the ability to work away from the instrument.

I was soon afforded an opportunity for more formal training in the art of mental imaging when I started auditioning again. Like many musicians, I am plagued by audition nerves that give me vibrato (wrong hand) and up-bow staccato (wrong time). Rather than using beta-blockers to conquer this problem, I went to my family doctor for training in self-hypnosis. The basic technique was quite easy to learn and I soon realized that mental imaging was a useful tool for many other aspects of my life, including power naps and practicing. One of the first exercises my doctor led me through involved mentally playing my audition concerto. I discovered that when I played it through in my mind, I always missed one difficult shift, so I had to begin reprogramming my mind to *hear* the shift correctly ("audiating," as opposed to visualizing). It took a few more attempts before I could imagine myself *playing* the shift correctly, actually feeling the fingerboard and string as if I were really playing. (Especially when you are just learning how to do mental practicing, it is easiest to do with music that you have memorized.) The next time I practiced the concerto, without consciously thinking about the shift that had given me trouble, I was amazed to find that I was able to get it right every time.

As I got better at self-hypnosis, I started to use it specifically to help with my practicing. I was really pleased with the progress in my playing and despite my long absence from work I was a better violinist than I had been before my injury. And like all skills, the more I used this ability to practice mentally, the more proficient I became. I have found it to be an invaluable resource that is woven into my practice pattern and takes no special effort at all.

Now, if I could just get rid of my right-hand vibrato at auditions. . . .

Note

1. Friedrich, Otto. *Glen Gould : A Life and Variations*.

Chapter 12

Working as an Athletic Musician

Work Protocols: Surviving Life as a Student or Working Musician

Getting through a workday or school day involves the same basic principles as getting through a day of private practicing. The difference is that in a practice situation you are in control of how, when and what you play, while in a working or student situation you must meet other people's demands.

Warming Up for Work

Warm up before a rehearsal or concert as you would before practicing at home, but if you feel a little self-conscious about breaking into your country line dancing routine at the rehearsal hall, you can do a few minutes of arm swings instead. Try warming up with a brisk walk – park your car a few blocks away from the stage door or get off the subway one stop too soon. I know a teacher who lives on the seventh floor of an apartment building who has her students take the stairs up to their lessons rather than the elevator. They arrive warmed up and ready to do their stretches before they play.

Stretching before Work

When you know you have a rehearsal or concert to play, you should make a special point of warming up and stretching thoroughly at home. When you arrive at work, go through the job-specific upper body stretches you need. (See Chapter 10.) These can be done anywhere, as the only special equipment you'll need is a doorway for the pectoral stretch.

Warming Up with the Instrument

Warming up with the instrument isn't a problem if you can arrive a few minutes before you have to play. Most musicians plan to arrive early for concerts, but rehearsals can find them rushing from one end of town to another, just managing to arrive in time to tune. If this is the case, you may be out of breath when you sit down to play, so the first step of your warm-up would already be complete. Try to incorporate onstage stretches at the beginning of the rehearsal (see below), and take advantage of the time it takes to get a rehearsal going to silently get your fingers moving on the instrument. Where possible, play a little less intensely for the first few minutes of the rehearsal than you might in the heat of a performance. Strings, for instance, can use a more relaxed vibrato and a minimum of pressure on the fingerboard.

Students should be given an opportunity to warm up before lessons start. If there isn't a place to play while you wait for your teacher, ask for a few minutes alone to go through your warm-up. Work with your teacher to ensure that the first part of your lesson is spent playing suitable "warm-up" material.

During Rehearsal

Surviving long working days does not mean coasting through rehearsals or concerts. Once you are warmed up, you should be able to play as intensely as you wish for the duration, but the more demanding the repertoire and schedule, the more careful you need to be about posture, stretching, and breaks.

Onstage Stretches

Stretching before and after you play is important. Developing the habit of stretching *during* rehearsals or concerts is good insurance against injury. When stretching is an integral part of your playing routine as well as something that you add in before and after, it is much less likely to be neglected. It also ensures that you change position regularly and take brief breaks from your work.

Many of the stretches and exercises that you have read about in Chapter 10 can be done on stage during a concert or rehearsal.

Pectoral Muscle Stretch

A doorway is the best way to perform this stretch. However, once you have mastered it you can stretch while seated, provided the chair back is the right height. Hook your arms over the back of the chair and gently lean forward. Hold 30 seconds. If you can't put your instrument down to do this, stretch one side at a time, being careful not to twist your spine (see photo 39, p. 148).

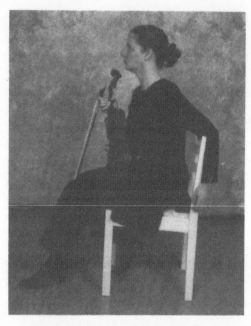

Photo 39. Onstage pectoral muscle stretch.

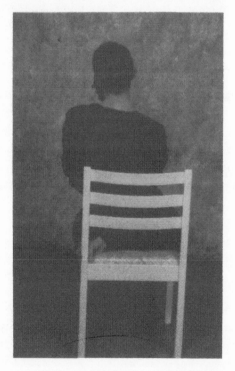

Photo 40. Onstage deltoid muscle stretch.

Deltoid Muscle Stretch

Slide to the back of your chair, reach behind with your right hand and grab the left edge of the chair seat. Bend gently to the left and hold. (It takes just a slight sideways motion to feel the stretch, so you can do this during a concert without anyone noticing.) Repeat on the other side (see photo 40, p. 148).

Forearm Muscle Stretch

With your wrist bent backward and fingers straight and supported by something (the music stand, the neck of your bass, etc.) push gently forward and hold for 30 seconds (see photo 36, p. 119).

You can also do this stretch by sitting on your hands with palms facing down, provided your arms are the right length! This is a very necessary stretch for pianists and can be done with both arms at once while seated at the piano bench.

The scroll stretch for violinists and violists is another variation on this theme. When you have a few bars' rest, turn your left hand away from you, putting the scroll between your first and second fingers. Gently push your wrist toward the scroll. Hold, and release. This stretches the forearm and wrist, and also untwists your arm (see photo 41, p. 150).

Forearm De-rotation Stretch

Violinists and violists who must keep their left arm rotated when they play need to untwist that arm periodically. You can de-rotate and stretch your left arm by sliding to the back of your chair, turning your hand clockwise, and grabbing the chair leg from behind. Hold 30 seconds (see photo 42, p. 150).

Neck Stretch

You can do neck extension stretches anywhere. They might look a little strange during a concert, but can certainly be done during rehearsals, in an orchestra pit, or while teaching (see photo 43, p. 150).

Onstage Exercises

Many of the exercises that you need to do on a daily basis can be done during rehearsals and concerts. You can totally incorporate them into your actual playing routine, as they can be done in time segments as short as an eight-bar rest. They can become as much a part of your playing as making reeds or rosining the bow. The only time you will need to make a point of doing them on their own

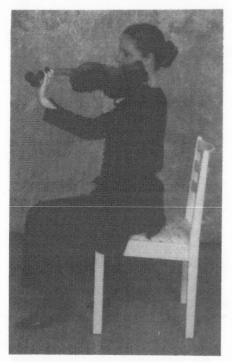

Photo 41. Onstage scroll stretch, left.

Photo 42. Onstage de-rotation stretch for forearm, right.

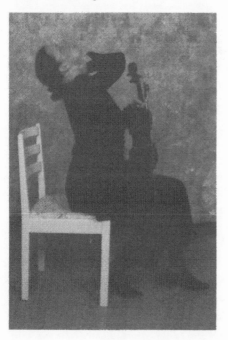

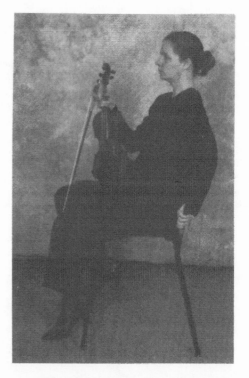

Photo 43. Left, rehearsal or pit neck extension stretch.

would be when you're on vacation.

Shoulder Rotator Cuff Muscles Exercise

If you are in a pit or at a rehearsal, take your elastic out and do a few exercises when you have a moment. If you are at a concert or are a little self-conscious about performing in public what many people misinterpret as bust development exercises, it is possible to get sufficiently proficient at this exercise to do it without the band. You won't get as much strengthening on each contraction, as you will be working without resistance, but if you can learn to push your elbows down and tighten the shoulder blade muscles isometrically, you can perform this imperceptible "twitch" hundreds of times throughout the day. (See photo 34, p. 113.)

Neck Retraction Exercise: The "Chicken"

This exercise fits easily into a few bars' rest. It can be done without using your hand. For full retraction without looking conspicuous as you apply over-pressure, you can cover your cheek with your hand as you use the heel of your palm to push your chin back. (See photo 44, p. 152.)

Back Extension Exercises

Percussion or bass players can do back extensions throughout any rehearsal or concert. Those of us stuck in a chair can do a seated variation of the back extension exercise by sliding to the front of the seat and putting one or both hands on the lower back and leaning backward over them. If you can, do five to ten repetitions at a time. These are also easily done during coffee breaks. (See photos 45 and 46, p. 152.)

Cool Down and Final Stretches

Ideally, we should all spend a few minutes at the end of rehearsals or concerts playing warm-up material, especially if we've just finished three hours of Bruckner or Mahler, etc. (This may not be necessary if your rehearsal has fizzled out gradually.) If you're in a big hurry to leave, spend just a few minutes on job-specific stretches, especially if you haven't included them during the rehearsal. It feels great to get out of that chair and do a few back extensions and stretches as you pack up, and you will leave in better shape to tackle your next rehearsal. (See photo 46, p. 152.) Look back through Chapter 10. Think like an athlete and be innovative – see which stretches and exercises you can adapt to fit the needs of your particular instrument and playing demands.

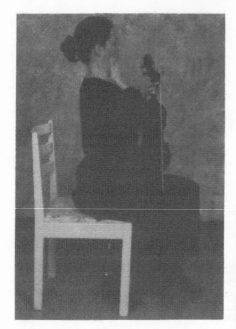

Photo 44. Onstage "chicken exercise" neck retraction with slight overpressure, left.

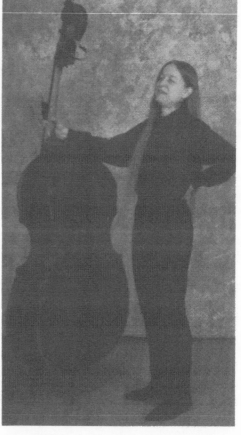

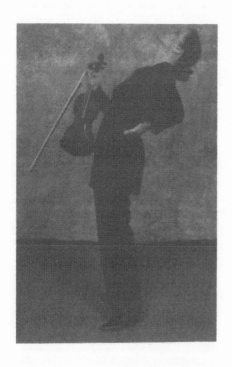

Photo 45 left, and photo 46 above. Back extension exercise, to do whenever there is a break in rehearsal or performance.

Chapter 13

The Work Environment

Many years ago, underpaid nurses were expected to work very long hours, often in poor conditions, without complaint. Dedication was supposed to be its own reward. Sadly, this philosophy still applies to many employed musicians. Few other professionals who really love their work would tolerate some of the working conditions that so many musicians face. Most nonmusicians, including medical practitioners who are treating musicians' injuries and advising musicians to be "sensible" about their work, often have no idea what the demands of our day-to-day life are and how little control we have over our work environment. While professional players have the protection of a union which puts some parameters on working conditions, there are still many things that are not or cannot be regulated. For instance, unions can control the length of a rehearsal and stipulate how breaks are scheduled, but this doesn't help a freelance player working triple-service days for various employers at once. And as musicians are not always their own best advocates, even working "union" jobs I have had to cope with four-hour dress rehearsals on concert days, Wagner operas (Wagner didn't belong to the AFM), extreme cold or heat, poor ventilation, noxious fumes, falling scenery, et cetera. Students may have an even more difficult time. Depending on their particular music school or summer program, they may find themselves scheduled for eight-hour days in various ensembles, as well as trying to keep up with their practicing. Hopefully, the day will soon come when administrations are more enlightened, but until then students must learn to cope as best they can.

There are many health issues other than injuries that are of particular importance to musicians. Each facet of music-making carries its own risks and musicians need to be aware of what these are. It's beyond the scope of this book to deal with these issues in detail, but here's a brief outline that might start you thinking and encourage you to be more vocal about improving working conditions.

Orchestral Playing

One of the biggest difficulties facing the orchestral player is having to sit down to play. If you play with the same orchestra all the time, explain to management the benefits of providing good chairs for injury prevention. The chair that you work in will not be the same as the chair that you relax in. Your chair should be the correct height for you, it should allow for movement and rest and, for most players, should have a forward sloping seat. When you have to make do with poor seating, do what you can to compensate. (See photos 48 and 49, p. 155.) Take advantage of scheduled breaks to get out of your chair. Our union *does* ensure that we get regular breaks, so be sure to use them to stand up and stretch.

String players should be aware of the advantages of rotating seating. Unlike winds, who usually don't share a stand and sit facing the conductor straight on, each different string chair will have its drawbacks. Sitting on the outside of the seconds, for instance, is one of the most uncomfortable spots for your neck – you need to turn one way to see your music and another to see the conductor. Alternating within a section and from inside to outside on a stand will vary your position. For violins, alternating between sections is helpful. First violins tend to spend more time in higher positions than the seconds, putting the left wrist in flexion more often. Seconds may have an easier time with their wrists, but are plagued by having to play so much on the D and G strings, overusing the deltoid. A similar situation would exist where there is a lot of divisi writing for the cello section, with outside players having to stress the deltoid by playing on the higher strings. If players and management both understood the benefits of seat rotation, perhaps the concept would be more universally accepted.

As you get involved in your playing, try to keep in touch with how your body feels. As was the case with my shoulder injury, the first warning signs of trouble often go unnoticed. In a concert situation, you may have to keep going even if you are in pain. (This shouldn't happen, so if you *do* experience pain during a performance, ice as soon as possible and make any appointment with a physiotherapist.) You can bear in mind an interesting phenomenon documented by sports psychologists:

"Muscular endurance and tolerance of fatigue related pain were enhanced when a physical task was performed conjointly with others as compared to solo performance."[1]

You can see why orchestral players get into trouble when you also consider that "When injury pain is relatively minimal and the attentional demands of sport [playing] are high, pain may be neglected, leading to increased injury risk especially for chronic overuse syndromes."[2]

Symphony musicians also need to ensure that their work environment does not put their hearing at risk. While decibel levels in a symphony orchestra will not remain as consistently high as they might in a rock band, they can peak at levels high enough to endanger hearing. This can be dependent on placement in the orchestra and the repertoire being performed. Noise-induced hearing loss is

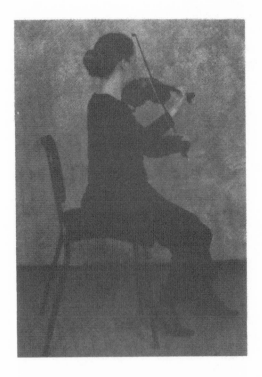

Photo 47. Demonstrating excellent sitting posture for playing, easily accomplished on Wenger Corporation's protoype "Stouffville Chair."

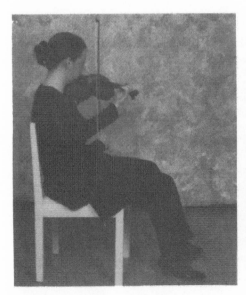

Photo 48. Poor posture playing on an inappropriate chair.

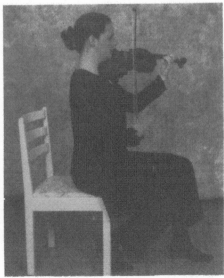

Photo 49. Making the best of a poorly designed chair.

irreversible and is often accompanied by tinnitus which can be very debilitating. Musicians and orchestra managements need to consider acoustically designed rehearsal facilities, noise barriers and personal hearing protection.

The Perils of the Pit

The main advantage I can think of to playing in a pit is that you can perform exercises and movements that wouldn't be acceptable on stage. The big drawback is that often there is so little room to move. Office workers would not put up with a workstation where they had to sit hunched or twisted to fit into the few square feet of space allotted to them, but pit musicians often tolerate this as "part of the job."

If you are a theater or opera/ballet musician who has an opportunity to get caught up with your reading during long breaks, be aware that unless you are very careful, your posture while hunched over that crossword on your knee is likely to hurt you more than anything you can do with the instrument. In the pit, unlike the concert stage, players are often able to keep drinks, books, equipment, etc., on the floor beside them. During the course of a rehearsal or show, notice how many times you bend over to pick small objects off the floor. Chapter 6 explains why repeated forward bending is dangerous, especially when coupled with lifting even light objects from a seated position. Many players attach a small shelf to their stand, like those used by reed players to hold their paraphernalia. This can save a lot of sustained back flexion. Despite using these shelves to hold their reed-making equipment, woodwind players, who are usually so diligent about posture when they play, often get into terrible positions when they start messing about with their reeds.

Safety in the pit is another big concern, especially for theater musicians. Sir Isaac Newton discovered the law of gravity long ago and anyone working in an orchestra pit knows that what is onstage does not always stay there. Most theater managements have yet to decide that safety netting is essential. Proportionately, overuse is responsible for far more injuries than accidents, but this is of small comfort to the injured musician, especially as accidents *can* permanently end one's career, or life.

Pit musicians face all the same risks to their hearing as orchestral players with the additional dangers of working in closer proximity to each other, and to amplified instruments.

The Hazards of Teaching

Many musicians develop problems related to poor posture when they teach. If you usually sit during lessons, you need to ensure that you have a decent chair and that you get out of it as often as possible. If you sit and write during lessons, you can find yourself developing neck problems from maintaining a head down and head forward position. See if you can rig up an inclined writing desk that will bring your work up closer to you (see photo 8, p. 59). Whether you are currently suffering through a neck problem or not, you may want to avoid writing altogether. I like to jot down fairly detailed practice instructions for my students, but I have also found that having the students write their own reminders can be effective. Taping the entire lesson is another possibility.

Standing to teach is fine if you can make sure that you are keeping your head up. If your pupils are very young, you may be constantly bending over to work with them. Have very short students stand on a plywood platform at their lessons.

Notes

1. Martens R, Landers DM: Coaction Effects on a Muscular Endurance Task: *The Research Quarterly* (1969), 40(4), 733-37.

2. Heil J: Psychology of Sport Injury: *Human Kinetics Publishers,* Box 5076, Champaign, Illinois. 1993.

Chapter 14

If You Are Injured

Where to Go for Help

Fifty years ago the health care scene must have been much simpler. Then a doctor was a doctor, a dentist was a dentist and a therapist was a physiotherapist or a psychoanalyst. Nowadays, you usually need to do a little investigation before accepting treatment or advice for your aches and pains. Many more options are open to you – but you do need to be sure that you are indeed getting the help you would prefer from the health care professional that you really wished to consult.

To add to the general confusion, the title "doctor" has now been adopted by many nonphysician groups. Originally, "doctor" indicated that this person had graduated from a university with a Ph.D. "doctorate," or from a university's faculty of medicine as a medical doctor (MD). (The Ph.D. groups seldom used their title, not wishing to confuse the public or be called upon in an airplane for a medical emergency.) This is no longer the case and the title "doctor" tells you very little.

"Therapist," alas, is now a meaningless title. There is no such academic qualification. Anyone can say they are a therapist. "Exercise therapists" probably like exercising. "Ergonomic therapists" probably like exercising and lifting weights with good posture – neither title is indicative of any formal qualifications. If you do your own housework you can call yourself a "home therapist."

So, ask your "doctor" and your "therapist" to give you more information. You need to know their precise qualifications as well as the direction of their postgraduate education. Physiotherapy in Canada became a bachelor of science qualification in the early seventies, so some older physiotherapists will have the earlier Dip.P.T. after their name. Those from England are M.C.S.P.s. Each country has formal initials which indicate qualified physicians and physiotherapists, and you should look for these on their business cards and on the diplomas hanging on their office walls. If you are in any doubt, call their respective colleges or a university and check out registrations, qualifications and unknown initials. The College of Physicians and Surgeons and the College of Physiotherapists are the regulatory bodies for these professions and are in the Yellow Pages. They can easily clarify if you're seeing the real McCoy.

Your next decision is whether you would prefer to consult someone who is part of orthodox medicine or someone who is part of "alternative health care." Orthodox medicine includes all health care professionals who graduate from university faculties of medicine or from schools affiliated with faculties of medicine. These include medical doctors, surgeons, dentists, physiotherapists, registered nurses, occupational therapists, speech-language pathologists and psychologists. No one will mind if you ask them to clarify this. It's not sufficient to ask them if they have a university degree as that degree could be in a totally different subject, such as business or engineering.

Kinesiologists, for instance, graduate with a B.Sc.Kin., but are not health care professionals. Many of them do become interested in the treatment of injured people when they are employed to lead exercise or fitness programs in clinics or hospitals. They must, however, return and graduate as a health professional before they are qualified to diagnose injuries or prescribe treatments. Some of the best orthopedic physiotherapists you will meet have taken that route, first studying normal human movement in kinesiology, then the problems induced by injury and pathology in medical or physiotherapy schools.

"Alternatives to orthodox medicine" includes just about everyone else who treats injuries. Examples are massage therapists, athletic therapists, chiropractors, naturopaths, reflexologists, shiatsu therapists and acupuncturists. Each have their own beliefs and philosophies and train in their own schools and colleges, but not in universities.

Occasionally, orthodox medicine and alternatives overlap. Many physicians and physiotherapists, for instance, have pursued acupuncture skills, using this as another tool for pain control. I have also met one chiropractor who had first qualified as a registered nurse and another who subsequently qualified as an MD.

Should you decide to consult an alternative health care provider, you can obtain further information about their education, philosophy, beliefs and treatments from their respective associations and colleges.

Only when armed with sufficient information should you decide to whom you will entrust your hurt body. As when choosing a tutor or teacher, you should have some basic expectations. Expect to be treated courteously, to be listened to and to have your injury carefully and thoroughly examined. Expect to have the problem explained to you very clearly, or to be referred to someone else for another opinion. Expect to be informed how to avoid seemingly endless treatments and how to prevent recurrences of the injury. Expect to feel progressively better with a treatment regime that will end in what you both agree is a reasonable length of time. If you and your doctor or therapist become old friends, you're probably going to the wrong one! (Christine has no choice – we work together.)

Playing through an Injury

If you have sustained a nonplaying-related injury, it may be safe or even preferable to continue playing through your injury. Playing-induced injuries, such as the various overuse injuries described in previous chapters, seldom recover if you continue to play with pain. By contrast, trauma injuries may be safe for gentle playing, within tolerable discomfort. In fact, with some activity, moderate sprains, strains and safe (stable) fractures usually heal faster and with better healing tissue than they would if they were immobilized.

Ask an orthopedic surgeon for advice about moving any part with a broken bone. Ask your physiotherapist how much to use a sprained or strained joint or muscle. All injuries are different and require individual rehabilitation protocols, so make sure your health professional clearly understands what you'd like to do. Their idea of moderate activity may not be the same as yours.

Christine's Two Cents' Worth

My shoulder story is a great example of what can happen when you continue to play with a painful overuse injury. Unless you've corrected the cause of the problem, you may find yourself in the same situation I did, where severe pain and loss of movement make it impossible to play. This was not the case with a more recent injury (a losing argument with an icy parking lot which resulted in a hairline fracture in one of the bones of my left hand). I was able to continue working, with Barbara's assurance that playing would not displace or disrupt the small, stable fracture in my hand. "Moderate activity" in this case meant less playing time, more frequent breaks and concentrating on bowing rather than strenuous left-hand playing. As fatigue limited the amount of time I could manage to play and I wanted to be able to keep my work commitments, I cut back on my own practice time and limited it to the sort of playing that normally constituted my warm-up. I also got reacquainted with my ice pack.

A car accident was my most recent (and hopefully final!) injury experience. It resulted in torn muscles and ligaments on my right side and as these take four to six weeks to heal, I had no choice about taking a month off work. As soon as I could, I began playing for short periods of time. With this injury, my left hand was okay, but I could bow only on the E string. I had to be careful with my warm-up too, as many of my usual stretches would have aggravated my injuries.

Depending on your instrument and the nature of your injury, you may be able to work to some degree wearing a supportive brace, or using equipment to help support the weight of the instrument. Adaptations to the instrument that are less than ideal on a long-term basis may prove worth doing while you recover. For example, a pianist could practice on an upright rather than grand piano, string players could use a lower bridge to reduce the amount of effort needed to depress the strings, etc. In my case, my whiplash injury meant altering the height and position of my shoulder rest and holding my head in a slightly different position from usual.

Regardless of what type of injury you are recovering from, spending time on mental practice, studying scores, listening to recordings, etc. can be really helpful and make the difference between depression . . . and severe depression! Fortunately, we heal.

Rehabilitation after an Injury

Anytime you are away from playing for an extended period of time, getting back in shape is not easy. Starting back after an injury is even more difficult, but I know from my own experience, and from Barbara's work with musicians who have gone through more horrifying sagas than mine, that it *is* possible.

Being given the green light to resume playing marks the beginning of a new struggle. If you've been unable to play for a long time, or if playing has hurt, the prospect of starting from the very beginning can be overwhelming. In fact, this is a time that many musicians make career changes. After successful rehabilitation of their injury, they may not be willing to face the prospect of starting over again with the instrument, especially if they have established an alternative career when they were away from music. For those who still want to get back to playing, knowing that it's possible can be a great encouragement and knowing how others have managed to do it can be helpful.

Recovering players seem to fall into two camps: the overdoers and the ones afraid to try. The majority fall into the first camp and Barbara has come to expect the phone call she gets a few weeks after she has "graduated" one of these enthusiastic musicians from the clinic. The once-injured musicians, having gone through a careful program of treatment and rehabilitation, arrive at the point where they can play pain-free and are so happy to be back at it that they go overboard and play their way back to an overuse injury. ("Overuse" is an understatement – there are some like the cellist, recently recovered from a long, severe bout with injury, who wondered why she hurt after playing 14 hours in one day!)

If you have had an injury that caused severe and prolonged pain, fear of the pain associated with your original injury and fear of re-injury may prove to be obstacles to your recovery. It can be difficult to distinguish between muscles protesting the end of a long vacation (which is not harmful and is to be expected) from true pain signaling *"Danger – Stop!"* Sports medicine teaches us that pain which is benign in nature generally does not persist after an activity, and is not accompanied by heat, swelling or increased tenderness. Harmful pain is usually sharp, occurring during activity and persisting for several hours after activity. It is usually accompanied by swelling and increased tenderness.

It can be difficult to distinguish the difference between discomfort that exists simply because you haven't played for a long time and discomfort that is signaling danger of re-injury. Just like the ballplayer at training camp, getting back to playing after a long break will feel strange and uncomfortable at first. If you think you can't start back because playing doesn't feel comfortable at the very beginning, you likely won't ever get back to playing. If you carefully follow a sensible training schedule, it won't take long before you feel stronger and more at home with the instrument.

The first few steps back can be slow and frustrating. It's hard to regain that feeling of ease with the instrument when you can play only five minutes a day, and you will feel as though you will never be able to play enough to regain your skills. Most of us do not truly appreciate how much physical effort it takes to play, or notice the necessarily strange postures playing puts us into, until we've been away from it for a while. Be patient – it will come.

Work with your physiotherapist to establish a training routine. Too much playing too soon can lead to re-injury, but fear of re-injury in itself can hinder your recovery. If you are feeling uncomfortable and tired after five minutes and are afraid to continue, stop playing, but try another five-minute session later in the day.

You may want to add a third or fourth session of the same length before you start playing more than five minutes at time. It can take a bit of trial and error, as you may push too much and set yourself back a step, or you might be too cautious and not progress. In my experience, once I received the right help, progress was steady, although not effortless and not without its ups and downs. I found the first few weeks of playing the hardest to cope with, both physically and emotionally, but once I made it over that hump it did get easier, and the progress I made was enough to inspire me to keep going.

Chapter 15

Stouffville Musicians' Physiotherapy Clinic

The Stouffville Musicians' Physiotherapy Clinic (see photo 50, p. 164) inhabits a century-old building on the main street of Stouffville, Ontario. This is a small, country town about 30 miles northeast of Toronto and its official title is Music Town, Ontario. For a musicians' clinic, it affords a quiet, relaxed and private location.

The Clinic is staffed by Maureen, our office manager, Susan, our fitness appraiser and myself, with Christine joining in as our consultant whenever this is requested by a musician. If we need more clinical help, physiotherapists from the parent clinic, York County Physiotherapy & Sports Injuries Clinic, bring their considerable expertise.

The Stouffville Musicians' Physiotherapy Clinic opened in 1991, and hurt musicians from all over North America have found their way to our door. Gradually, the staff is expanding, as other musicians who recover from their injuries and are interested in what they have learned offer their services as consultants for their own particular instruments. We have decided that this close partnership between a clinician and a musician who understands functional anatomy is the essential ingredient for successful results.

Much to my surprise, the fact that I am not a musician (but do appreciate music) has been a help rather than a hindrance. No one minds playing for me once they realize that I have no preconceived ideas about how they should play and will simply be watching what playing does to the body. Most musicians soon realize that their talent delights and amazes me, so they relax and give good demonstrations of their habitual playing postures and positions. Over the years they have also patiently taught me about their instruments and common problems.

Christine and I have discussed this gradual overlapping of our knowledge bases many times. Although we find each other's disciplines fascinating and continue to learn as much as possible from each other, when dealing with problems of injured musicians in the clinic, our roles remain distinct.

Clients attend initially for an hour's consultation with me. Violinists and violists may then, if they wish, spend another hour with Christine, experimenting with her growing collection of chin rests and shoulder rests and occasionally

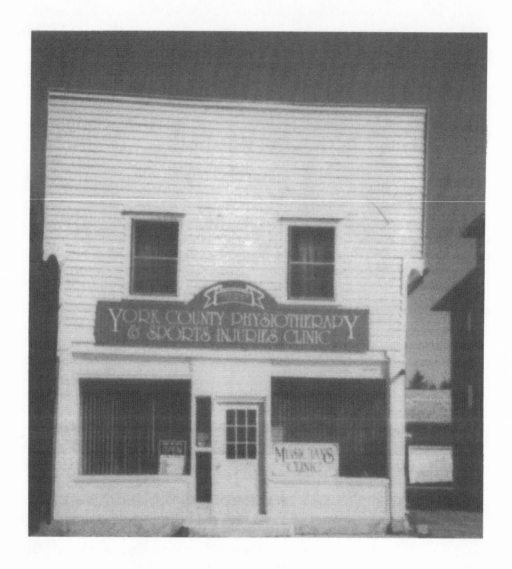

Photo 50. The Stouffville Musicians' Clinic.

photographing or videotaping until we all are satisfied with the changes. The musician then goes off to try all the exercises, stretches and changes we have suggested. Some only need that one visit. A few need to return a few times until we all are satisfied with the results. Most will telephone us or respond to Maureen's "mother hen" calls to tell us how they are doing.

For a few who need a course of injury-specific physiotherapy treatment, this can usually be arranged at a clinic close to home – especially for students who generally need a government-funded facility. So far we have been pleased with the results, but where do we go from here?

Glancing back to the first chapter of this book with its alarming injury statistics, both collected and suspected, it seems obvious that we should be concentrating our energies upon "prevention" as well as "cure." Injury prevention is an inherent component of physiotherapy and Christine is equally determined that musicians should be spared her miserable experiences. To address this, in 1992 we designed a one-day injury-prevention workshop for musicians, titled "Playing Without Pain." During the workshop we impart much of the information contained in this book, and conduct practical sessions which include practicing many of the recommended stretches and exercises. Christine then demonstrates corrective ergonomics, using volunteers who are looking for ways to improve their playing postures.

We have presented the workshop to many groups of musicians and to some of their physiotherapists. (See Appendix.) Invariably, it has been received with enthusiasm and a sense of relief that "something can be done." Group discussions usually continue right out into the parking lot or to a local restaurant.

We have also ventured outside of Canada, presenting papers at international medical conferences in Hong Kong, Australia, and England. (See Appendix.) Here we learned that the problems of musicians' injuries are indeed widespread. We also soon realized that the chief reason for the rather sparse help so far provided by orthodox medicine appears to be due to the fact that the majority of physicians and physiotherapists are unaware that there is a major problem.

Many of them are also musicians, with a genuine appreciation for music. Few of them, however, play sufficiently to induce overuse playing injuries as they are busy with their clinical practices, so they lack firsthand experiences to draw upon. And, as mentioned previously, few hurt musicians consult them. No wonder those who do specialize in this field feel rather alone.

However, our presentations were received with great interest and enthusiasm. In Australia, this led to discussions with local musicians and management groups, all actively searching for effective injury prevention and rehabilitation. Hopefully these medical and musical people will now get together and change the course of these injuries. In Canada, musicians continue to attend our workshops and the majority report that they can decrease their pain and manage their injuries more successfully when they have a better understanding of the underlying causes and simple preventive techniques.

Many music teachers who have participated have delighted us with their positive responses. Once they have been exposed to basic anatomy and athletic protocols, many can hardly wait to try out these new ideas with their pupils and to give us the benefit of their own experiences and experiments (see photo 51, p. 167.) Music teachers, in our opinion, are the main line of defense against playing injuries for the generations to come. If they are willing to incorporate our teaching into theirs, the Stouffville Musicians' Physiotherapy Clinic should eventually run out of injured musicians to treat.

Nothing would make us happier!

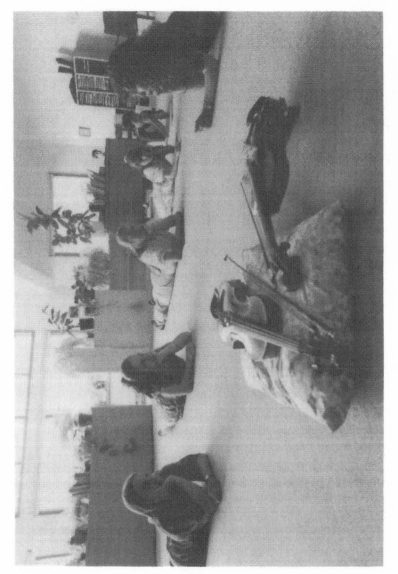

Photo 51. The music teacher. This music teacher is incorporating injury prevention into her program at a Chamber Music Day Camp.

Glossary of Terms

Alexander technique - a school of exercises, posture and movement.
articular cartilage - smooth covering of the bone ends within a joint.
biceps - muscle on the front of the upper arm that bends the elbow and turns the hand palm up.
bursa - soft, fluid-filled sac or cushion.
bursitis - inflammation of a bursa.
carpel tunnel syndrome - compression of a nerve to the hand at the wrist level.
chicken and egg syndrome (C&ES) - confusion or indecision about which came first.
deltoid - main shoulder muscle that lifts the arm.
dermatome - area of skin that derives feeling from a nerve.
disc - the cushion between spinal bones.
ergonomics - the study of how to work efficiently and safely.
Feldenkreis - a school of exercises and movement.
flexion - bending forward.
humerus - bone in the upper arm.
impingement - nipping or squeezing.
impingement syndrome - pain experienced due to nipping of soft tissue.
infra spinatus muscle - one of the rotator cuff muscles, stabilizing the shoulder.
labrum - fibrous cuff around the socket of the shoulder joint.
ligament - strap that holds a joint together.
lordosis - normal curve in the low back and neck.
mental practicing - recreating physical practicing in your imagination.
muscle - strong, elastic tissue responsible for moving our joints.
muscle imbalance - one set of muscles moving a joint has become over-strengthened.
nerve - the brain's communication line with the body.
orthopedics - pertaining to the treatment of disorders of bones and joints.
overuse playing injury (OPI) - injury caused by stressing part of the body beyond its tissues' physical endurance level.
passive treatment - any treatment done to one by someone else.

pelvic tilt - flattening the low back curve and tucking in the buttocks.

physiotherapy - the assessment, diagnosis, management and prevention of injuries and movement disorders.

protocol - regimen.

protraction - moving the head and neck forward ahead of the body, horizontally.

repetitive strain injury (RSI) - same as OPI.

retraction - moving the head and neck backward on the body, horizontally.

rotator cuff muscles - muscles connecting the shoulder blade and the head of the humerus.

scapula - shoulder blade.

sciatic nerve - large nerve running from the low back down the leg to the foot.

sciatica - pain down the leg caused by pinching of the sciatic nerve.

service - term used by musicians to describe any period of work.

shoulder impingement syndrome - see impingement syndrome.

soft tissue - muscles, tendons, ligaments, capsules, nerves, discs, etc. - everything we're made of except bones and teeth.

spinal cord - bundle of nerves extending from the brain down through the spine.

supra spinatus muscle - one of the rotator cuff muscles.

swayback - faulty posture, in which one is leaning backward from the waist, overaccentuating the low back curve.

tendon - strong band or cord of tissue connecting fleshy part of muscle with bone.

tendonitis - inflammation of a tendon or tendon sheath.

teres minor muscle - one of the rotator cuff muscles.

thoracic inlet syndrome (TIS) - compression of nerves to the arm at the base of the neck.

thoracic outlet syndrome (TOS) - same as thoracic inlet syndrome.

tinnitus - a sensation of ringing or buzzing in the ears.

triceps - muscle on the back of the upper arm that straightens the elbow.

vertebra - spinal bone.

visualization - calling up a distinct mental picture of something previously seen.

warm-up - gentle activity designed to prepare the body for strenuous work.

Appendix

What's Been Done and Said

"Playing Without Pain" is an innovative workshop program dealing with injury prevention and management for musicians. Barbara Paull and Christine Harrison designed this program in 1992 and have presented their workshop to musicians in various venues, including:

> Sir William Osler Health Care Centre
> University of Western Ontario
> Niagara Youth Orchestra
> State University of New York, Buffalo
> University of Toronto (combined Faculty of Music/Faculty of Medicine presentation)
> Chamber Music Day Camp, Thornhill
> American String Teachers Conference, Rochester
> The Royal Conservatory of Music, Toronto
> University of Toronto, Settlement House
> Huron Heights Secondary School, Newmarket

Seminars have been presented to health professionals at:

> York County Hospital, Newmarket
> Oakville/Trafalgar Memorial Hospital
> Soldier's Memorial Hospital, Orillia
> Women's College Hospital, Toronto

The following are samples of direct quotations from written evaluation by participants:

"Beautifully and clearly presented . . . I wish someone had reached me with your message when I was 20. I especially appreciate the exercises you demonstrated – I know they will make a difference to me."
> Olga van Kranendonk, Cellist, Tafelmusik

"This should be a mandatory course for all musicians, especially those involved in the teaching of our next generation of artists . . . Fabulous – Perhaps the most important information I've ever been given."
B. Morrison, Pianist and Teacher

". . . (Christine's) story is wonderfully inspirational . . . encouraging to see that there is real help now available to deal with these problems."
Leslie Knowles, Violinist, Toronto Symphony Orchestra

"Your unique collaboration of a professional musician who has been through it all and a concerned, registered therapist resulted in a practical workshop of inestimable value to students, teachers, and symphony musicians alike . . . preventative medicine at its best."
Dr. Robert Skelton, Professor of Violin, University of Western, Ontario

"A wonderful workshop – a huge amount of the material can be directly related to problems I see with my flute students on a daily basis."
Margot Onodera, Flute Teacher/Performer, Royal Conservatory of Music, Toronto

". . . one of the most valuable presentations we have ever had for our students . . . indispensable to anyone aspiring to play and teach a string instrument."
Ralph Aldrich, Professor of Viola, University of Western, Ontario

"Once again you have rewarded us with a most informative workshop that has stimulated our clinical enthusiasm. Christine was able to clearly demonstrate habitual postural malalignments that facilitated our grasp of the neck-shoulder relationship."
Sandra Bates, B.Sc. P.T., Oakville - Trafalgar Memorial Hospital

"I've never been to a more fun or interesting workshop in my life!"
12-year-old string player, Niagara Youth Orchestra

"What a terrific workshop you presented for us. We heard so many positive comments about it like – the 'best ever!' Your approach was very clear, extremely well organised and informative for all."
Muriel Bodley, Vice-President, National School Orchestra Association

"One of the most informative and practical sessions I have attended . . . in over 30 years . . . As a non-musician, I had to attend a music clinic to learn how

to sit at my desk/computer and alleviate my shoulder pain."
      Edward Eagan

      Barbara Paull and Christine Harrison have presented papers on the subject of musicians' injuries at the Science and Art of Physiotherapy International Conference, Hong Kong (1993), the 12th World Congress of the International Federation of Physical Medicine and Rehabilitation, Sydney, Australia (1995), the 1st World Congress in Neurological Rehabilitation, Newcastle-upon-Tyne, England (1996) and Health and the Musician, 1st International Conference, York, England (1997).

References

Caldron PH, Calabrese LH, Clough JD, et al.: A survey of musculoskeletal problems encountered in high-level musicians. *Med Probl Perform Art* 1:136-39, 1986.

Cyriax J: Textbook of Orthopaedic Medicine, Volume l, 5th edition. *Bailliere Tindall*, London 1969.

Cyriax J: Textbook of Orthopaedic Medicine, Volume ll, 8th edition. *Bailliere Tindall*, London 1971.

Elvey RL: Brachialplexus Tension Tests and the Pathoanatomical Origin of Arm Pain. In Idczak IM (ed): Biomechanical Aspects of Manipulation Therapy. *Lincoln Institute of Health Sciences,* Carlton, Australia. 1981.

Fishbein M, Middlestadt SE, Ottati V, et al.: Medical problems among ICSOM musicians: Overview of a national survey. *Med Probl Perform Art* 3:1-8, 1988.

Friedrich O: Glen Gould: A Life and Variations. *Lester & Orpen Dennys,* 1989.

Fry HJH: Prevalence of overuse (injury) in Australian music schools. *Br. J. Ind. Med.* 44:35-40, 1987.

Green B, and Gallwey WT: The Inner Game of Music. *Doubleday.* 1986.

Heil J: Psychology of Sport Injury: *Human Kinetics Publishers,* Box 5076, Champaign, Illinois. 1993.

Janda V: Altered Patterns of Recruitment of Skeletal Muscles: Recognition and Correction. 1991.

Kopandji IA: The Physiology of the Joints. Volumes 1 & lll. *Churchill Livingston.* 1974.

McKenzie RA: The Cervical and Thoracic Spine. Mechanical Diagnosis and Therapy. *Spinal Publications Ltd.* New Zealand. 1990.

McKenzie RA: The Lumbar Spine. Mechanical Diagnosis and Therapy. *Spinal Publications Ltd.* New Zealand. 1981.

Maitland GD: The Slump Test. *Australian J.P.T.* 31:6, 1985.

Mandal AC: The Seated Man. *Dafnia Publications.* Denmark. 1985.

Martens R, Landers DM : Coaction Effects on a Muscular Endurance Task: *The Research Quarterly* 40(4), 733-37, 1969.

Nachemson AL: The Lumbar Spine, an Orthopaedic Challenge. *Spine* 1:59-71, 1976.

Newmark J, Lederman RJ: Practice doesn't necessarily make perfect: Incidence of overuse syndromes in amateur instrumentalists. *Med Probl Perform Art* 2:142-44, 1987.

Pratt RR, Jessop SG, Niemann BK: Performance-related disorders among music majors at Brigham Young University. *IJAM* 1(2):7-20, 1992.

Ramazzini B: Wrote in 1713 "No sort of exercise is so healthful or harmless that it does not cause serious disorders . . . when overdone."

Reid DC: Sports Injury Assessment & Rehabilitation. *Churchill Livingston.* 1992.

Twomey L, Taylor J: Flexion Creep Deformation and Hysterisis in the Lumbar Vertebral Column. *Spine* 7:2:116-12, 1982.

Twomey L, Taylor J: Age Changes in Lumbar Intervertebral Discs. *ActaOrthop. Scand* 56:496, 1986.

Wyke B: The Neurology of Low Back Pain. Ed. Jayson M.I.V. *Pitman Medical Ltd.* Tunbridge Wells. 1980.

About the Authors

Barbara Paull, M.C.S.P., M.C.P.A., physiotherapist

Barbara Paull is a British-trained registered physiotherapist who immigrated to Canada in 1967. She has concentrated on orthopedic physiotherapy in many different clinical settings for over thirty years. In 1985 she left York County Hospital in Newmarket, Ontario, where she had been director of physiotherapy, to open her own clinic also in Newmarket. In 1992 she opened a second clinic in Stouffville, Ontario, dedicated to musicians. Presently Barbara is a consultant, clinician, and lecturer in orthopedic physiotherapy. She has presented papers on musicians' injuries in Australia, England, the United States, Canada and Hong Kong. She is copresenter of the injury prevention workshop for musicians, "Playing Without Pain." Barbara lives in the country north of Toronto with family, many animals, a temperamental septic tank, and a very good-natured husband.

Christine Harrison, violinist

Christine Harrison is a freelance violinist working in Toronto, Canada. She has performed with various symphonic, chamber, and theater groups, including work with the Canadian Opera Company, the Hamilton Philharmonic Orchestra, Amadeus Ensemble, and productions including "The Phantom of the Opera," "Miss Saigon," and "Sunset Boulevard." In addition to her performance career, Christine has extensive experience teaching violin. Her interests in the field of musicians' injuries have resulted in her role as string consultant to the Stouffville Musicians' Clinic. She is copresenter of the "Playing Without Pain" workshop for musicians.

175

Made in the USA
Lexington, KY
06 April 2013